Greco-Roman Medicine and What It Can Teach Us Today

Greco-Roman Medicine and What It Can Teach Us Today

Nick Summerton

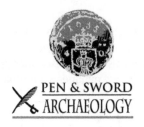

PEN & SWORD
ARCHAEOLOGY

First published in Great Britain in 2021 by
Pen & Sword Archaeology
An imprint of
Pen & Sword Books Ltd
Yorkshire - Philadelphia

ISBN 978 1 52675 287 1

Printed and bound in the UK
by CPI Group (UK) Ltd, Croydon, CR0 4YY

Pen & Sword Books Ltd. incorporates the Imprints of Pen & Sword
Archaeology, Atlas, Aviation, Battleground, Discovery, Family History,
History, Maritime, Military, Naval, Politics, Railways, Select, Transport,
True Crime, Fiction, Frontline Books, Leo Cooper, Praetorian Press,
Seaforth Publishing, Wharncliffe and White Owl.

For a complete list of Pen & Sword titles please contact

PEN & SWORD BOOKS LIMITED
47 Church Street, Barnsley, South Yorkshire, S70 2AS, England
E-mail: enquiries@pen-and-sword.co.uk
Website: www.pen-and-sword.co.uk

or

PEN AND SWORD BOOKS
1950 Lawrence Rd, Havertown, PA 19083, USA
E-mail: uspen-and-sword@casematepublishers.com
Website: www.penandswordbooks.com

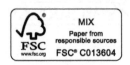

MIX
Paper from
responsible sources
FSC
www.fsc.org   FSC® C013604

Contents

List of Plates

Acknowledgements

In developing this book, I am indebted to many individuals stretching back over thirty years. However, I should like to express my particular thanks to Dr Ralph Jackson who has never lost patience with my many questions, providing me with a wealth of information and contacts in addition to facilitating my access to the collections at the British Museum. I am also very grateful to Heather Williams and Yuen Ting Baker at Pen & Sword Books for their support and encouragement in bringing this project to fruition.

Others have generously provided me with illustrations, resources and guidance. Many of these individuals are mentioned both in the preface and elsewhere within the text. However, I should especially like to thank Lord Bledisloe for permitting me access to the site at Lydney on several occasions, as well as to Martin Jones and Sally Pointer for all their superb work on the Roman reconstructions.

Above all, I must express my enormous gratitude to my parents, Barry and June, my wife, Ailie, and my three daughters, Katrina, Siân and Emily, for accompanying me on my numerous forays in search of the Greco-Roman world. Katrina also helped me to design the front cover alongside Jon Wilkinson.

Preface

Some elements of this book started life as a short work for Shire Publications entitled *Medicine and Health Care in Roman Britain*. In the conclusion I wrote that:

> *it would be wrong for us to dismiss the Roman approach to health care and to assume that we have got it entirely right today. Nowadays, many patients who consult their general practitioner are suffering from symptoms that are often due to the stresses and strains of modern life. Over-investigation of such somatic symptoms as fatigue, dizziness or headaches can cause considerable harm. Suggesting that such patients spend a quiet week resting, bathing and taking occasional brisk walks with the dogs in a place such as a Lydney [a Romano-British healing sanctuary] would, perhaps, be of greater benefit.*[1]

This final paragraph really marked the start of a long journey leading to the present book. In addition to seeking to better understand the Roman approach to health care, I wanted to consider what it can still teach us today. Also, although I have retained some of my earlier focus on Roman Britain, there has been a significant expansion to consider, in greater detail, the consequences of being part of the wider Roman Empire.

Over the last fourteen years I have had the privilege to meet or to correspond with several experts who have been enormously generous with their time and advice in specific areas. John Wilkins explained how he had adapted Galen's ideas on hygiene for today's world. Adrian Harrison was instrumental in my initial forays into reconstructing some ancient eye remedies. Bryn Waters encouraged a greater focus on the locations and the activities at ancient healing sites in the UK and elsewhere. Melinda Letts kindly supplied me with access to her fantastic work on Rufus of Ephesus including a translation of *Quaestiones medicinales.* Onora O'Neill helped me to look afresh at our current medical regulatory systems and to re-examine the writings of Scribonius Largus, and John Ratcliffe's work on Celsus and ancient surgery provided significant new insights.

In parallel, I continued as a general practitioner, clinical epidemiologist and public health physician, roles that helped me to look at Roman medical practice from a variety of perspectives. This has also enabled me to reflect on some less positive aspects of modern developments in health care, most importantly the adverse consequences of regulation in distorting or, in one tragic case, destroying good clinical practice.

CHAPTER 1

Introduction

There is a wealth of excellent modern literature exploring various aspects of Greek and Roman Medicine. In writing this book, I have consulted numerous texts and doctoral theses, in addition to a raft of papers in peer-reviewed journals. However, the vast majority of such publications focus on studying ancient medicine for its own sake without considering any practical benefits that might have relevance today.

It is always important to respect the autonomy of the past in terms of the differences in material culture as well as the dissimilar ideas, priorities, hopes and fears of our forebears. But I do not believe that this should be a barrier to drawing inferences, ideas or lessons with a view to examining our current approaches to health and wellbeing. Finding ways to cope with disease, death, disability and distress have been constant concerns throughout all human history.

There can be little doubt that the Romans experienced many of the illnesses that are still encountered today. Individuals would also have had to decide how best to deal with their health-related concerns. Nowadays, some patients might consult their doctor as soon as they experience back pain, but most are more likely to use a home remedy, discuss it with a close friend or relative, visit the pharmacist or even consider a complementary therapist. Similarly, although the range of treatment opportunities would have been different for the Roman patient, individual choice would still have played an important part in determining the type of care selected.

In considering any aspect of ancient medicine, it is crucial not to become blinkered by a modern perspective; health and health care must always be seen in context. For example, a condition considered 'normal' in one society (or at one time) might represent a medical problem in other circumstances. Currently in the UK, low blood pressure is generally not treated but elsewhere in Europe the situation is different. *Jambes Lourdes* is a common condition in France but unrecognised in most other countries. Furthermore, illnesses that warrant the input of a doctor nowadays might, at other times, have been very effectively dealt with by other healers.

In examining Roman medicine, a particular challenge is the enormous time frame. The departure of the last Western Roman emperor, Romulus Augustus, in AD 476 marked over 1200 years since the foundation of Rome. In the east it then continued for another 1,000 years as the Byzantine Empire. A further issue is that there was significant hybridisation of Roman institutions and beliefs with many other ancient cultures. For example, the medicine being practised during the period when the Romans occupied Britain was essentially an amalgam of theories and practices derived from the indigenous inhabitants of Rome, the Etruscans, the Egyptians and the Greeks, combined with the pre-Roman local health beliefs prevalent before they arrived.

An Egyptian haematite amulet has been found within a Roman context near Welwyn in Hertfordshire. It is inscribed with a representation of the uterus, a scarab beetle and the name '*Ororiouth*', a protector spirit against women's diseases.[2] At Bath, the presence of the haruspex Lucius Marcius Memor suggests Etruscan influences on medical care. Haruspication involved slaughtering an animal, usually a sheep, and then carefully examining and 'reading' the liver and intestines. It was believed that specific aspects of the health of the person bringing the sacrifice could be determined from the anatomy of the animal's internal organs.[3]

In Roman Britain and elsewhere, the Greek impact on Roman medicine was particularly dominant and writings by Greek-born physicians such as Galen and Dioscorides continued to be studied and used in Europe for over 1,300 years after the demise of the Western

2

Roman Empire. Also, most doctors recorded on inscriptions from Italy and the Western Latin provinces of the Empire before AD 100 bore Greek names.

Therefore, this book focuses on Greco-Roman medicine as it might have been practised during the *Pax Romana,* a 200-year period commencing with Augustus and concluding with the death of Marcus Aurelius. Moreover, each main chapter – preventive medicine and the preservation of health, healers and patients, architecture and health, pharmaceutical remedies, psychological wellbeing and holistic care, surgical and physical therapies – is subdivided into two distinct elements.

First, an attempt is made to reconstruct the Roman context drawing on the ancient literature supplemented with evidence from archaeology, paleopathology, epigraphy and numismatics. A second section then reflects on the Roman achievements highlighting some issues that might have continuing relevance today.

Although I have harnessed ancient literature to construct a window into the medical past, questions might be raised about the potential biases of the sources used. The physician Galen was a prolific author but has also been categorised as opinionated, verbose and arrogant. The natural historian Pliny the Elder is sometimes considered insufficiently critical of the masses of information he collected and, in relation to Celsus, it remains unclear whether he was a physician or just a very careful observer. To address such concerns I have avoided, as far as possible, undue focus on a single author or an exclusive concentration on medical writings.

Any attempt to re-construct and interpret the past is also at risk from an author's selective use of selected sources together with an occasional drift into nostalgia.[4] Therefore, in drawing inferences I have largely avoided focusing on precise problems as opposed to considering some broader health care concerns such as the balance between prevention and care, the relationship between healers and patients, trust and regulation, and the role of technology. Only in relation to pharmaceutical remedies does the discussion take a different turn in accordance with the experimental archaeological findings. As pointed out by John Tosh, history presents us with a range of alternatives that might be considered when faced with a particular situation.[5] There is always more than one approach to dealing with any predicament so, perhaps, a menu of options from past experiences can help us today.

Clearly there will always be a requirement to continue to exercise extreme caution in drawing any lessons from the distant past. But, by rigidly adopting a twenty-first-century view, it is also all-to-easy to dismiss or denigrate some aspects of ancient medicine and yet to overplay others significantly. How can we be confident that a bronze instrument was an effective surgical tool? Did our medical ancestors make important therapeutic advances or were most of their treatments simply working as placebos? Are aqueducts, drains and bathhouses really a reflection of the Roman concern for the public health? Should we simply dismiss dream therapy or pilgrimages to healing sites as gimmicks? Is there any real value in listening to patients – or even to meet them face-to-face – to make a diagnosis or a prognosis? As we continue to cope with the coronavirus pandemic can we learn anything from the Roman response to their ancient plagues? I hope this book will serve to answer these questions and many more besides.

CHAPTER 2

Preventive Medicine and the Preservation of Health

The Romans and their doctors attached a great deal of importance to following a particular lifestyle (termed 'regimen', 'hygiene' or 'dietetics') with a view to maintaining health. The second-century physician and author Galen made a specific distinction between the preservation of health when it is present (hygiene) and the restoration of health when it is affected by disease (therapeutics).[1]

Galen's six books on the preservation of health, *De sanitate tuenda* (*Hygiene*), were written around AD 175.[2] In addition to drawing from the Greek doctor Hippocrates' works *Regimen in Health*, *Regimen I*, *Regimen II*, *Regimen III* and *Airs, Waters, Places*, Galen also considered the writings of Diocles of Carystus, Praxagorus of Cos, Herophilus of Chalcedon, Erasistratus, Asclepiades of Bithynia and Theon of Alexandria in crystallising his ideas.[3]

Prior to Galen, several Greek philosophers including Empedocles of Acragas developed the doctrine that all matter within the universe – including human bodies – was a mixture of four elemental substances (fire, air, water and earth) and four elemental qualities associated with them (hot, cold, wet and dry). Linked to this, it was determined that the human body contained four humours – blood (hot and wet), yellow bile (hot and dry), black bile (cold and dry) and phlegm (cold and wet).[4]

It was believed that the four humours needed to be in the correct amounts and strengths for a body to be healthy. The proper blending and balance of the four humours was known as '*eukrasia*'. Imbalance of humours – or '*dyskrasia*' – led to disease. In general, illness was

5

about the excess or the lack of a specific humour or the exacerbation of one quality over another (hot or cold; dry or wet).[5]

Importantly, humours were not considered to be present in equal quantities in everyone. Therefore, a physician wishing to re-balance an individual's humours had to consider a number of factors such as a person's lifestyle, age and temperament in addition to the season.[6]

To the Greeks and the Romans, health was something that existed in its own right and was not simply the absence of disease. According to Galen, health was *'that state in which we neither feel pain nor are impeded in the functions pertaining to life'*. And *'That which is in accord with nature. Disease is that which is contrary to nature.'*[7]

In 'accord with nature' was taken to mean a situation in which the body was in perfect balance in relation to seven 'naturals'.[8]

1. The four elements – air, fire, earth and water
2. The four qualities – hot, dry, cold and moist
3. The four humours – blood, yellow bile, black bile and phlegm
4. The different parts (members) of the body divided into
   a. The fundamental (brain, heart, liver)
   b. The subservient (nerves, arteries, veins)
   c. The specific (bones, membranes, muscles)
   d. The dependent (stomach, kidneys, intestines)
5. The faculties (energies) – natural, spiritual and animal
6. The spirits – natural, vital and animal
7. The functions (operations) of the body – hunger, digestion, retention, expulsion

Galen also recognised that *'the range of health is very wide and not exactly the same for all of us'*,[9] adding that *'one must not determine those who are healthy and who are diseased simply on the basis of the strength or weakness of the functions; one must apply the term "in accord with nature"'*.[10] In addition, he made the important point that a problem affecting the body might be '*so small and imperceptible as not to disturb those who have it*'.[11]

Hygiene was about seeking to restore the status quo thereby preventing disease and preserving health. In a book written for Thrasybulus, Galen proposed that hygienic measures should be targeted at three groups: those who appear healthy already, those who are recovering from an illness and those who are in an intermediate state between heath and illness (e.g. the elderly or individuals experiencing fatigue).[12]

The priority was to identify the factors under some degree of human control that could facilitate or obstruct the power of nature (sometimes referred to as the 'non-naturals').[13] For example, the first century philosopher Seneca wrote that:

> *it is quite contrary to nature to torture one's body, to reject simple standards of cleanliness and make a point of being dirty, to adopt a diet that is not just plain but hideous and revolting. In the same way as a craving for dainties is a token of extravagant living, avoidance of familiar and inexpensive dishes betokens insanity.*[14]

The medical hygienist's goal was to maintain the normal equilibrium of humours and qualities by recommending the correct kind and amount of, for example, food, drink, sleep, wakefulness, sexual activity and exercise. In *Ars medica (The Art of Medicine)* Galen outlined the key elements to consider in developing a healthy regimen as:

> *one from association with the ambient air, another from movement and rest of the whole body and its parts, a third from sleeping and waking, a fourth from those things taken in, a fifth from those things excreted or released, and a sixth from the affections of the soul.*[15]

The first five items on Galen's list (i.e. air, movement, sleep, diet and excretions) will be considered in greater detail within this chapter and the sixth, affections of the soul (psychological wellbeing), is the focus of Chapter 6. Certain physical therapies such as massage, bathing, phlebotomy and rocking were often part of the hygienic regimen too,[16] and these are covered in Chapter 7.

It was also seen as extremely important to tailor the approach to individuals taking into account age, gender, lifestyle, constitution, co-morbidities and place of residence. In addition, there was a requirement for balance between the various components of a hygienic regimen and to ensure that a person was not under-emphasising or over-emphasising any specific element. Galen wrote:

For just as it is impossible for cobblers to use one last for all people, so too it is for doctors to use one plan of life that is beneficial to all. Because of this, then, they say it is most healthy for some to exercise sufficiently every day, whereas for others, there is nothing to prevent them passing their lives wholly in idleness. Also, for some it seems to be most healthy to bathe, whereas for others it does not.[17]

In addition Galen sought to consider the realities of people's lives within his writings commenting: '*that there are very many differences of the bodies themselves, in the same way there are also very many kinds of lives we lead*'.[18]

Air

Pure air was particularly important to the Romans and Galen recommended avoiding air tainted by marshes, industrial processes, odours from drains or rotting remains. He was keenly aware of atmospheres that were '*stifling and foul, analogous to the air in houses that are shut up in which mould collects due to putrefaction and lack of ventilation. Such airs are harmful for all the stages of life*'.[19] The first century author Celsus advised his readers to reside in a house that is *'light and airy'*[20] and the lawyer Pliny the Younger, emphasised the gentle breezes and the healthiness of the *'clear sky and the pure air'* at his Tuscan villa.[21] He also commented on the design of his Laurentine villa allowing *'the western breezes to enter and circulate'* so that *'the atmosphere is never heavy with stale air'*.[22]

Smoke and fumes from the burning (or the partial burning) of carboniferous fuels for cooking or heating must have been a major problem for the Romans. It has been suggested that so many fires were lit across the Empire it caused a level of air pollution that cooled the European climate at the time.[23] Seneca commented that

> *no sooner had I left behind the oppressive atmosphere of the city and that reek of smoking cookers which pour out, along with the cloud of ashes, all the poisonous fumes they've accumulated in their interiors whenever they're started up, than I noticed the change in my condition at once.*[24]

In addition to affecting the levels and the balance of humours, air was relevant to two other important facets of ancient physiological theory – *pneuma* and *innate heat. Pneuma* was an ethereal substance derived, in part, from inspired air and circulated around the body enabling the key organs to function. Once it reached the rete mirabile at the base of the brain, a psychic *pneuma* was produced that was responsible for consciousness, sensation and voluntary movement.[25]

Originating in the heart, *innate heat* supported the vital functions of the human body. Over the course of a person's life it gradually lost strength being eventually extinguished on death. According to Galen, it was *'preserved by the occurrence of moderate exercise, not only of the body but also of the mind'*.[26] Fresh air was seen as important in helping the *innate heat* to maintain its equilibrium especially by cooling.[27]

Based on a comparative study of ancient literature and the archaeological remains of the gardens at Pompeii, it has been proposed that the Roman idea of 'pure air' and health should be characterised broadly in terms of sensations and associations. Thus, the Romans might have recognised 'pure air' by the feel of a gentle breeze; the sounds of moving air, wildlife or water; light or sweet aromas as well as natural sights and colours especially blue, green and white.[28]

Movement

According to Galen *'for the preservation of health, exertions must come first, followed by food and drink, and next in order, sleep, and then sexual intercourse for those who intend to engage in this'*.[29] He also made it clear that any movement could only be termed exercise or exertion if it brought about a change in breathing.[30]

Celsus stated that *'useful exercises are: reading aloud, drill, hand-ball, running, walking; but this is not by any means most useful on the level, since walking up and downhill varies the movement of the body'*.[31] In addition to offering general advice on movement, Galen suggested specific exercises for different parts of the body, writing

> there are those that work out the loins more, or the arms, or the legs, and in other cases the whole spine, or the chest alone, or the lungs. In fact, walking and running are exercises specific for the legs, acrocheirism and shadow boxing are specific for the arms, bending forward and backward continuously for the loins. [32]

He also recommended taking very deep breaths or emitting very loud sounds to exercise the lungs. His views on sexual activity as exercise were that it was really designed for those in *'their prime'*,[33] but, subsequently, he indicated that men at all ages should *'keep an eye on the use of sexual intercourse – whether it is harmless for them or harmful to those using it'*.[34]

As will be discussed further in Chapters 4 and 6, healing sanctuaries, bathhouses and hospitals might have been located or designed to facilitate movement. The Roman architect Vitruvius was a particular advocate of the health benefits of exercise, explaining that *'in walking the body is heated by motion, the air extracts the humours from the limbs'*.[35] Some buildings even displayed images of exercising or athletes such as the so-called 'bikini girls' mosaic from the Villa Romana del Casale in Sicily. On this mosaic several Roman women are shown engaged in various sports: one carries weights, a second is about to throw a discus, two are depicted running and another pair are playing a ball game (Plate 1).

As with all hygienic interventions, Galen emphasised that one size does not fit all:

> *Experience shows that some people are harmed and some are benefited by the same things ... I know of some who immediately became sick, if they remain three days without exercise, and others who continue indefinitely without exercise and yet are healthy.*[36]

He went on to suggest that tailored exercise programmes might sometimes be required stating:

> *there were some whom I prevented from exercising at all, even with those exercises that are suitable, wishing them to be satisfied with the activities of life only. Some, however, I ordered to set aside the majority of exercises, so as to reduce the totality of exercise to a minimum. Some I directed to change the qualities only, or the order, or the time. Some, however, I directed to change their whole form of exercise.*[37]

Galen classified exercises by speed and vigour and, in common with Celsus, highlighted the importance of integrating exercise with other hygienic components including massage, bathing, food, and rest.[38] There was also an interaction between movement and air with Celsus writing that *'it is better to walk in the open air than under cover; better under the shade of a wall or of trees than under a roof'*.[39]

Galen also encouraged a consideration of 'opposites' to maintain the humoral balance suggesting that '*if the body has laboured too much on the previous day, do this by reducing the amount of exercises; if it has laboured too little, do this by increasing the amount of exercise*'.[40] Taking into account an individual's age also mattered, and, for older people, Galen recommended starting with a massage (with oils) followed by a gentle walk and some passive exercises.[41]

Both Galen and Celsus expressed concerns about people adopting the exercise regimes of elite athletes rather than integrating movement into their day-to-day activities. Celsus wrote: '*the example of athletes should not be followed, with their fixed rules and immoderate labour*'[42] and Galen added that '*better are rowing, digging, reaping, javelin throwing, running, leaping, horse-riding, hunting, fighting with heavy arms, chopping wood, lifting and ploughing, and all other things done naturally; these are better than exercising in a wrestling school*'.[43]

In his short book *De parvae pilae exercitio* (*On Exercise with a Small Ball*), Galen claimed that activities carried out with a small ball are the best. His rationale underlying this assertion was that it was easy to do, could be undertaken individually or in company, presented the opportunity to exercise all, or parts of, the body, could be tailored to different ages and constitutions and, above all, it was safe.[44] He also recognised the health benefits of travelling in a horse-drawn carriage due to the passive exercises linked to being shaken around.[45]

Sleep

Ensuring sufficient sleep – neither too much nor too little – was a key element of hygiene. It was recognised that there was a need to use the waking hours productively and to allow a period of calm in the transition between activity and sleep. The Romans knew that while it was natural to be awake during the day and asleep at night; pain, distress, psychological problems, symptoms of some physical ailments such as indigestion, or old age were common causes of insomnia.

To Galen, the more active the mind during the day, the better the chances of a good night's rest as the brain required sleep to recover. To help to get to sleep Galen recommended exercise, food and wine in addition to '*washing the head with copious hot baths*'.[46] Silence and fresh air were also invaluable aids to sleep as were occasional herbal treatments. There is evidence that lavender-filled pillows, chamomile drinks and lettuce (see Chapter 5) were all used by the Romans to treat insomnia.[47]

Seneca recommended a nightly confessional, in which he pleaded his case before his own tribunal:

Sextius had this habit, and when the day was over and he had retired to his nightly rest, he would put these questions to his soul: 'What bad habit have you cured today? What fault have you resisted? In what respect are you better?' Anger will cease and become more controllable if it finds that it must appear before a judge every day. Can anything be more excellent than this practice of thoroughly sifting the whole day? And how delightful the sleep that follows this self-examination — how tranquil it is, how deep and untroubled, when the soul has either praised or admonished itself, and when this secret examiner and critic of self has given report of its own character! I avail myself of this privilege, and every day I plead my cause before the bar of self. When the light has been removed from sight, and my wife, long aware of my habit, has become silent, I scan the whole of my day and retrace all my deeds and words. I conceal nothing from myself, I omit nothing. For why should I shrink from any of my mistakes, when I may commune thus with myself? 'See that you never do that again; I will pardon you this time ... In the future, consider not only the truth of what you say, but also whether the man to whom you are speaking can endure the truth.'[48]

Oversleeping was also seen as 'against nature' and for those wishing to languish in bed the Emperor Marcus Aurelius wrote:

> *At day's first light have in readiness, against disinclination to leave your bed, the thought that 'I am rising for the work of man'. Must I grumble at setting out to do what I was born for, and for the sake of which I have been brought into the world? ... to carry out Nature's bidding?*[49]

Diet

In terms of diet Celsus wrote that '*a surfeit is never of service, excessive abstinence is often unserviceable; if any intemperance is committed, it is safer in drinking than in eating. It is better to begin a meal with savouries, salads and such-like*'.[50] He also recognised that food and drink '*are of general assistance not only in diseases of all kinds but in preserving health as well*'.[51] To the Romans, adequate food and drink were vital to good health but the focus needed to be on those things that promoted health, strength, longevity and nourishment.[52]

Celsus divided foods into three groups according to their overall characteristics. In the top class he placed bread, pulses, the meat from large game and large domesticated animals, large birds, 'sea monsters' (including whale), honey and cheese; in the middle category smaller game, birds, fish and pot herbs whose roots or bulbs were eaten; and, at the bottom, vegetables, fruit, olives, snails and shellfish.[53]

Galen attributed certain imbalances of humours and qualities to consuming particular items. Foods and drinks producing excessive heat included onions, garlic, leeks and '*old or bitter wine*'.[54] The Hippocratic text *Regimen in Health*, the foundation for much of Galen's work on food and drink, advised people that, in winter (to balance the humours and qualities), they should eat as much as possible and drink as little as possible and that all meat eaten in winter must be roasted. As spring comes on, individuals could gradually drink more and move towards boiled meat rather than roasted, so that by the time of summer all meats are boiled.[55]

But, in achieving balance, the seasons were not the only aspect that mattered. Regimens had to vary according to an individual's constitution, habits and body type. Flabby individuals were advised to keep to 'dry' foods for most of the year to counteract the natural moistness of their qualities. In terms of habits, it was seen as dangerous to suggest a foodstuff, or a quantity of food, with which they were not familiar.[56] Any diet also needed to take into account a person's age and, for infants, Galen wrote that '*mother's milk is very likely best*'[57] but that '*wine is most undesirable, so for old men it is most useful*'.[58] Achieving a balanced diet was a very complicated process!

Eating cooked food rather than raw food, and in particular bread and meat, was viewed as something that set the ancient Greeks and Romans apart from animals and other peoples. Further 'cooking' was considered to take place in the body using the person's *innate heat*. Food was thought to begin its transformation in the mouth before undergoing additional changes in the stomach and liver until it eventually became blood; a process termed concoction.[59]

Irrespective of the comments of Galen and Celsus, it has often been assumed by many modern authors that the diet of the average Roman was monotonous and unhealthy. However, recent evidence derived from an examination of the mineral content of bones from Herculaneum in addition to bioarchaeological finds from the town's sewers is challenging this view.[60] The people living in the apartment block that fed into the Cardio V sewer, for example, seem to have consumed 114 different foodstuffs including 7 types of cereals, 12 varieties of fruit and 45 species of fish.[61] It seems increasingly likely that the diet of the population in Herculaneum at the time of the eruption of Vesuvius was healthy and mineral rich containing high levels of seafood and vegetable protein.

Towards the end of the first century Plutarch, the philosopher and essayist, expressed concerns that Romans no longer suffered from the diseases of want and deprivation but were now beset with diseases of luxury.[62] Seneca also wrote how he became

> *enthusiastic about keeping the appetites for food and drink firmly in their place ... I came to give up oysters and mushrooms for the rest of my life (for they are not really food to us but titbits which induce people who have already had as much as they can take to go on eating – the object most desired by gluttons and others who stuff themselves with more than they can hold – being items which will come up again as easily as they go down).[63]*

It is also interesting to note that some Roman cookbooks from the time began to include medical recipes to aid digestion;[64] perhaps to help some individuals cope with the increasingly rich fare. Scenes including food, drink, banquets, cooking, hunting and fishing are also favoured images on numerous Roman mosaics and wall paintings across the Empire.

In the Roman world, assessing if a person had an ideal body composition did not depend on measurements of height and weight but rather looking at an individual and determining if they were somewhere around '*the midpoint between being lean and having excessive flesh*'.[65] Fat people wanting to become thin were advised to eat '*only one full meal a day*', or to dine immediately after exercise.[66] More specifically, Pliny the Elder, the writer and natural philosopher, advised that those '*who wish to reduce themselves, or prevent the bowels from being relaxed, should abstain from drinking while taking their meal*'.[67]

Although the detailed dietary advice offered by the ancient authors is often complex, frequently confusing and sometimes contradictory, Galen neatly sums up his overall approach in a single sentence: '*the objective in respect of the nature of the foods and drinks in terms of quantity, quality and capacity is here again moderation, so as not to take too much or too little*'.[68]

Galen also made an important point that: '*I do not consider it right for a doctor to be completely ignorant of the art of cooking, because whatever tastes good is easier to digest than other dishes which may be equally as healthy.*'[69] In a separate essay, he even details the preparation of barley soup starting from the selection of the best barley and water right through to its use in the correct individuals.[70]

Excretions

It was thought that the unusable residues of concocted food and drink (superfluities) produced in different parts of the body would lead to humoral imbalances. There were three points of excretion: the rectum for dry/solid superfluities, the urinary bladder for wet/liquid superfluities and the skin for wet and vaporous superfluities through sweat and imperceptible transpiration.[71]

Dietary adjustments and exercises were often recommended to manage individuals with retained superfluities. Some people were also purged by, for example, phlebotomy, bathing (to encourage sweating), the use of laxatives or eliciting vomiting. Later Galenic theory held that if the 'natural seed' was kept too long in the body it would turn into poison, leading to the view that sexual intercourse was an important part of good health.[72]

One other aspect of excretions related to self-monitoring of bowel habits and micturition. For example, both Celsus and Galen recommended that individuals check the appearance of their urine each morning.[73]

What can the Romans teach us today?

In 1724 George Cheyne wrote *An Essay of Health and Long Life* and, in this, he acknowledged the debt to the classical world: '*as the ancients are not so frequently read, the advantage of modern works, which do not contain a single idea that is new, is to place before us useful truths that have been forgotten*'.[74]

But, despite the growing number of excellent translations, it still remains challenging to unearth the treasures that lurk within the classical texts. To Galen the purposes of the various hygienic measures were to keep the *krasis* of the body and its parts within the normal range (i.e. ensuring the appropriate mixture of humours and qualities), to maintain an acceptable level of *innate heat*, to preserve satisfactory levels of *pneuma* and to regulate the amount and nature of the superfluities arising from concoction within the body. Unfortunately, to modern doctors such ancient theoretical underpinnings are both confusing and make little scientific sense, leading some to abandon their quest to learn anything useful from Galen's writings.[75]

However, I would suggest that many of the practical hygienic recommendations from our ancient forbears have continuing relevance today. It is certainly hard to fault the advice from Galen and Celsus on movement or Seneca's and Marcus Aurelius' comments on sleep.

Hygiene in the twenty-first century

Towards the end of the second century AD, the Empire was devastated by the Antonine Plague. The effects of this illness – probably smallpox – were dramatic and it is estimated that it led to at least 5 to 10 million deaths. In some areas it might have killed as many as one-third of the population and weakened the Roman army for a generation.[76]

Galen encountered the plague at several points in his career. During a visit to Aquileia on behalf of the Emperor Marcus Aurelius he wrote:

> *the plague attacked more destructively than even before, so the emperors fled immediately to Rome with a small force of men. For the rest of us, survival became very difficult for a long time. Most, indeed, died, the effects of the plague being exacerbated by the fact that all of this was occurring in the middle of winter.*[77]

At the start of this decade, no doctor alive had encountered anything along the lines of our Antonine forebears. But as I write this chapter – in

18

December 2020 during the second wave of the coronavirus pandemic – over 65,000 people in the UK have died of the disease and the longer-term impacts on the wellbeing of the British population and the economy are difficult to assess.

However, it is worth reflecting that the Antonine Plague was much deadlier than coronavirus, and the society it hit was far less capable of saving the sick than we are today. But Rome continued, its communities rebuilt, and the survivors even came to look back nostalgically on the period of the plague as a golden age.

There were few reliable drug treatments available to Galen, so, in dealing with individuals with smallpox, his focus would have been on a person's general health and wellbeing based on the principles of hygiene. Keeping healthy is always important but even more so when our bodies might be asked to fight off a serious illness and there is certainly much to be recommended in Galen's approach to protect ourselves from the consequences of coronavirus. Individuals who are unfit, overweight or smoke will fare much worse if they should, unfortunately, catch the disease.

Throughout this year, I have certainly echoed Galen in emphasising to my patients the importance of getting outside every day for some fresh air and exercise. Walking in sunshine will also increase our vitamin D levels and this can help to boost immunity. In addition, I have talked much more about maintaining a balanced diet and avoiding overeating or drinking too much alcohol. I have also pointed out that smoking (and breathing in second-hand smoke from others) delivers poor air directly into the lungs.[78]

More generally, there is a growing body of evidence linking the quality of the air that we breathe to our wellbeing. In the UK we now spend more than 85–90 per cent of our time indoors and, aside from increasing our risks of catching coronavirus, poor ventilation in homes is also associated with asthma, allergic conditions due to house dust mites and sick building syndrome. But there are simple things we could all do to help, such as opening windows, watching out for damp and moulds and reducing sources of indoor air pollution from open fires, candles, smoking, aerosols, air fresheners and cleaning products.[79]

The cereals, fruits and vegetables being eaten in Herculaneum were more nutrient dense than is the case nowadays. Also, the residents of Herculaneum ate considerably more fish than are consumed by the area's population today.[80] Currently, across the whole world significant numbers of people still exist on diets that are deficient in whole grains, fruits, vegetables and seafood, something that might be compounded by a poor focus on nutrition in most modern medical training programmes.[81]

The Mediterranean diet, which started to be promoted from the 1980s, has a number of similarities to that enjoyed by the inhabitants of Pompeii and Herculaneum. Those following this regime consume more olive oil, legumes, unrefined cereals, fruits and vegetables. There is also a greater emphasis on fish than meat but people are restricted to only a moderate intake of dairy products and wine. Moreover, research has demonstrated that the Mediterranean diet has health benefits in terms of decreased risks for developing conditions such as cancer, heart disease and diabetes.[82]

Today, focusing on our excretions is still of great relevance to preserving health. Galen pointed out that a problem affecting the body might be *'so small and imperceptible as not to disturb those who have it'*[83] and that *'for the doctor, when inquiring ... to ask the patients themselves about everything that has happened to them'*.[84] In relation to the earlier diagnosis of cancer, for example, it is important to be alert for blood in the urine or stools; changes in the frequency of bowel movements or micturition; or excessive sweating.[85] Echoing Galen, the key thing is for individuals to be aware what is 'normal for them' and to respond if there are any changes that are 'not in accordance with nature'.[86] Celsus also emphasised the importance of self-awareness: *'everyone should be acquainted with the nature of his own body, for some are spare, others obese; some hot, others are frigid'*.[87]

Galen stated that *'health is a kind of balance'*[88] and, ideally, nowadays this should be about focusing on individuals alongside populations; about being aware that lifestyle and prevention as well as treatment all matter in preserving health; and about considering all the various facets of hygiene. Unfortunately, we still tend to be blinkered by specific risk factors such as blood pressure or cholesterol rather than considering an individual's overall chances of developing conditions such as heart disease or strokes. Many lifestyle interventions also seem to focus on altering a single aspect of human behaviour such as exercise, diet or psychological wellbeing rather than adopting a comprehensive approach.[89] Tailoring is also important: for example, just because you reach a certain age does not mean that you should stop exercising.[90]

As will be discussed in Chapter 3, self-sufficiency and looking after your own were fundamental Roman values. Galen made the point that *'the objective of hygiene is for us to take it upon ourselves to preserve health'.*[91] Celsus also commented that:

A man in health, who is both vigorous and his own master, should be under no obligatory rules, and have no need for a medical attendant, … His kind of life should afford him variety … but more often take exercise.[92]

The problem is that following Galen's principles of hygiene and focusing on the six 'non-naturals' can be very hard work.[93] During the late middle ages, many individuals certainly preferred the quick results of purging or bleeding to correct their excesses and, today, some of us would probably opt to simply swallow a pill while resting on the sofa in our warm homes. Worryingly, a recent study has shown that individuals at risk of strokes or heart diseases who have been put on medicines to lower cholesterol or cut blood pressure are actually more likely to become physically inactive and gain weight.[94]

Within the UK, lifestyle-related conditions arising from smoking, alcohol misuse, inactivity, obesity and poor diets are becoming a major concern. In 2010, 7.4 per cent of the population had been diagnosed with type 2 diabetes and this is expected to rise to 10 per cent by 2030. There are also now more than 3,000 alcohol-related admissions to accident and emergency departments every day.[95]

To compound matters, not all doctors are as lean and fit as they could be, setting a poor example to their patients. Galen was an exemplar, stating that:

after I reached the age of twenty-eight, having persuaded myself that there is an art of hygiene, I followed its precepts for the whole of my subsequent life, and was never sick with any disease apart from the occasional fever.[96]

John Wilkins and Christopher Gill at the University of Exeter Classics Department have sought to adapt Galen's ideas on hygiene for today's world.[97] In their first study they focused on six issues for maintaining wellbeing:

- Considering the food and drink consumed
- Ensuring the right amount and kind of exercise
- Living and working in an environment that is conducive to health and wellbeing
- Getting the right amount of sleep
- Actively caring for mental wellbeing
- Achieving a balance between all the above five factors. As discussed earlier, Galen did not develop a 'one size fits all approach' but tailored the regime to individuals.

The Exeter Galenic lifestyle programme was followed by fifty people over a two-week period during February 2012, with questionnaires and workbooks subsequently being completed. Of all the outcome measures used, including cumulative physical and mental wellbeing, a substantial majority of the participants registered a significant improvement in comparison with a control group.[98]

Another approach to hygiene with a particular emphasis on psychological wellbeing and termed the 'therapeutic lifestyle programme', has been developed by Stephen Ilardi at the University of Kansas.[99] His six factors are: sleep hygiene, social support, exercise, bright light exposure, dietary omega-3 fatty acid supplementation and anti-rumination strategies. In a small evaluation of the effectiveness of this approach, it was found that participants in the treatment group showed a significantly greater decrease in depressive symptoms, something that was maintained for at least six months.[100]

The hygienic Roman garden

Private gardens were popular with the Romans and over 500 have been discovered in Pompeii and Herculaneum. Under the Roman Republic, they were primarily designed for growing vegetables but, during the imperial period, many evolved into much grander affairs. Peristyle gardens became popular in town houses and these were well-lit decorative spaces adorned with flowers, herbs, water features and various types of statuary. At Ostia there is also evidence of a shared garden serving the residents of an apartment block. In addition, public gardens were sometimes developed in association with theatres, temples and bathhouses.[101]

Recently, I became involved in developing a new garden at the Roman site of *Isurium Brigantum* (Aldborough) in North Yorkshire. This furnished me with a fantastic opportunity to explore the Roman concept of hygiene as it might have been applied to their gardens.

The core products from Roman gardens were fruit, vegetables and herbs plus, on occasion, honey and wine. A wide range of plants were also available to the Romans and Pliny the Elder listed seventy cultivated for food or cooking, thirty-nine used for making wines or cordials and sixteen grown to encourage bees.[102] In addition, he mentioned 101 items with medicinal properties such as lettuce to help with sleep.[103] He also wrote how his research had been

aided by Antonius Castor, who in our time enjoyed the highest reputation for an intimate acquaintance with this branch of knowledge. I had the opportunity of visiting his garden, in which, though he had passed his hundredth year, he cultivated vast numbers of plants with the greatest care. Though he had reached this great age, he had never experienced any bodily ailment, and neither his memory nor his natural vigour had been the least impaired by the lapse of time.[104]

There is an overlap between the different purposes of plants (and plant-related products) with items, such as bay laurel or honey, having both culinary and medical uses (see Chapter 5). However, aside from providing medicinal plants and herbs, Roman gardens probably had a broader hygienic role in encouraging movement and enabling access to fresh air in addition to enhancing psychological wellbeing (see Chapter 4). In terms of the four elements (air, fire, earth and water), gardens might even be viewed as providing access to sunshine (fire), air, the sights and sounds of water in addition to landscapes and contacts with nature (earth).

From personal experience, I can confirm that significant physical work is involved in establishing and maintaining a Roman garden and, in his list of exercises, Galen specifically advocated *'digging, bearing burdens, pruning vines and reaping'*.[105] But it is also clear that established Roman gardens were designed to encourage movement both around the perimeter and in between the individual beds. Pliny the Younger described tree-lined pathways and avenues edged by box hedges at his villa in Tuscany.[106] Garden paths have also been identified archeologically from a number of villa sites including Frocester Court.[107] The Roman architect Vitruvius even provided details on the construction of sand-covered walkways or *ambulationes* incorporating drains and a charcoal base to ensure the surface remained dry.[108] Garden furniture including seats, tables and dining couches are found at many sites, presumably giving walkers chance to rest and view the garden.[109]

At Hadrian's Villa in Tivoli there is a large open structure enclosing a garden with a central pool (*Poikile*). The north wall has a double portico with circular turning points at both ends incorporating an inscription stating the distance covered by walking alongside the wall. This ambulatory wall might even have been specifically orientated to ensure that one side provided shelter and warmth on winter walks with the other face offering shade during the hot summer months.[110] Pergolas with shaded walkways were often included in Roman gardens and this is something that has been incorporated within the design at Aldborough.

To ensure fresh air many town gardens were placed at the rear of houses away from street odours. Pliny the Younger emphasised the views, breezes and smells at his garden villas including commenting on a '*terrace scented with violets*'.[111] The Aldborough garden site certainly receives fresh breezes and enjoys uninterrupted views towards the White Horse and the Yorkshire Moors beyond. Planting with scented plants including camomile, lavender, rosemary and roses also accords with the Roman approach.

Enabling psychological wellbeing (affections of the soul) was the sixth element of Galen's approach to hygiene and is discussed in greater detail in Chapter 6.[112] Although it seems likely that much of the heavy manual work involved in Roman gardening would have been undertaken by slaves, there is now good research evidence for the positive effects of any gardening in reducing anxiety, depression, stress and rumination (brooding), in addition to enhancing self-esteem.[113]

Gardening is also about being in contact with nature and, as well as the flora, the Romans encouraged birds into their gardens as evidenced by bird baths and feeders. Fishponds and, occasionally, aviaries have been identified at a several sites and some Roman gardens were adorned with fresco paintings showing greenery, flowers, birds and blue sky. There is also a growing body of evidence for the benefits of natural settings for enhancing psychological wellbeing.[114]

The coronavirus pandemic has demonstrated the significant adverse impacts on many people's mental health as a result of social isolation and I am sure this must have been the case for some of our predecessors too during the time of the Antonine Plague. But, as I have experienced at Aldborough, gardens and gardening are an excellent way to connect with others in a safe space outdoors and, for the Romans, they also served as areas for dining, conversation and worship.

CHAPTER 3

Healers and Patients

Some Roman patients might have had access to a physician, but many would have turned to a variety of other individuals to help with their health problems such as root cutters, gymnastic trainers, dream interpreters, eunuchs, boxers, grooms, pharmacists, midwives and priests.

Pharmacists (including those who made [*unguentarii*] or sold [*seplasiarii*] ointments) were widespread across the Empire and probably occupied an important place in supplying patients with remedies. A limestone stela from Rome shows a female pharmacist with a book resting on her knee and surrounded by numerous barrels and circular objects. Behind her are two colleagues; one is shown adding materials to a vat and the other is stirring the mixture. A fragment of a writing tablet found in a first-century military ditch at Carlisle refers to an '*albano seplasario*' and one of the numerous Vindolanda writing tablets mentions another pharmacist, Vitalis.[1]

In considering the medical services available to the Romans, it is important to be particularly careful in applying our modern labels. For example, Pliny the Younger wrote to the Emperor Trajan about a healer who had saved his life:

Last year, Sir, when I was in serious ill-health and was in some danger of my life I called in an iatralipten, and I can only adequately repay him for the pains and interest he took in my case if you are kind enough to help me. Let me, therefore, entreat you to bestow on him Roman citizenship.[2]

But it is unclear whether Pliny's *iatralipten* was a physical therapist, ointment doctor or masseur.

For many traditional Romans, the concept of a personal professional physician was an anathema. It was at odds with the Roman values of self-sufficiency and looking after your own. On some Roman farms, it seems that the head of the household (*pater familias*) enjoyed the role of chief healer with responsibility for the health of his family and any estate workers. The Roman agriculturist and farmer Varo wrote: '*There are two divisions ... in the treatment of human beings: in the one case the physician should be called in, while in the other even an attentive herdsman is competent to give the treatment.*'[3] One of the Vindolanda writing tablets suggests that the women of military families were sometimes expected to deal with the day-to-day health problems that arose in their households and kept a selection of medicines to hand for this purpose. In letter 294, Paterna wrote to Lepidina: '*I shall supply you with two remedies*', one of which was for fever.[4]

Many aspects of Roman culture and society were strongly influenced by the Greeks and their impact on Roman medicine was particularly dominant. The earliest recorded reference to Rome's interaction with Greek medicine occurred in 293 BC when, according to the Roman historian Livy, the god Aesculapius arrived in Rome in the form of a snake. Rome had experienced three consecutive years of plague and, after consulting the Sibylline Books, an embassy was dispatched to Greece seeking divine medical assistance. Subsequently, a temple to Aesculapius and an associated healing complex, were established on Tiber Island [Plate 2].[5]

Around seventy years later, the Greek physician Archagathus migrated to Rome from the Peloponnese and was asked to stay. According to Pliny the Elder:

citizen rights were given him, and a surgery at the cross-way of Acilius was bought with public money for his own use. They say that he was a wound specialist, and that his arrival at first was wonderfully popular, but presently from his savage use of the knife and cautery he was nicknamed 'executioner' and his profession, with all physicians, became objects of loathing.[6]

These comments by Pliny – together with those of others at the time – illustrate the Roman distrust of the Greek influence on medicine.[7] But, despite these initial misgivings, Greek physicians flocked into Rome, encouraged, to some extent, by Julius Caesar's offers of citizenship and tax immunities for medical practitioners.[8] Soon, the Romans were adopting many Greek healing practices in addition to assimilating their medical vocabulary into Latin.

Physicians

When the Emperor Claudius crossed the English Channel in the early days of the Roman invasion of Britain, he was accompanied by at least two doctors: Gaius Xenophon and Scribonius Largus. Xenophon, Claudius' personal physician, was subsequently given the title praefectus fabrum; another honour lavished on this rather ungrateful doctor who, according to the first-century Roman historian Tacitus, eventually helped Claudius to his end: '*while pretending to help Claudius to vomit, he put a feather dipped in a quick poison down his throat. Xenophon knew that major crimes, though hazardous to undertake are profitable to achieve*'.[9]

Other emperors, governors and men of substance were attended by personal physicians who would often travel with them. During one imperial progress, Apollinarus, physician to the Emperor Titus, even commented on a successful visit to the toilet in Herculaneum, by scratching on the wall the words: '*Apollinaris medicus Titi Imp; hic cacavit bene.*'[10] The Emperor Septimius Severus, who is said to have suffered badly from gout, certainly had two doctors in attendance upon him during his Scottish campaign. On the return of the Emperor to York, the physicians received instructions from the Emperor's son, Caracalla, that they should hasten the death of Septimius Severus. Their refusal was disastrous for them and it is possible that their remains are among the beheaded skeletons unearthed at York in 2005.[11]

There is epigraphic evidence for the presence of physicians right across the Roman Empire. Moreover, numerous inscriptions from the west, including Britain, indicate that around two-thirds of doctors were Greek or of Greek descent. For example, two altars written in Greek and dedicated by doctors have been found in Chester[12] and another physician of Greek extraction was practising at Binchester.[13] The Chester inscriptions are translated as:

To the mighty Saviour Gods, I Hermogenes a doctor set up this altar

[Plate 3]

The doctor Antiochus honours the all-surpassing saviours of men among the immortals. Asclepius of the gentle hands, Hygeia and Panakeia

[Plate 4]

Both altars were found within the area of the military fortress and near a building whose design resembles that of a legionary hospital (see Chapter 4). The text on the altar by Antiochus was particularly poetic, perhaps an attempt to emphasise his educated status. But, whether either Hermogenes or Antiochus were legionary doctors, civilian doctors or, perhaps, personal physicians to senior officials remains uncertain. Intriguingly, Hadrian's personal physician was also called Hermogenes.

Across the Empire there is evidence of female doctors such as Flavia Hedone (Nimes, France), Matilia Donata (Lyon, France), Julia Saturnina (Emerita, Spain) and Sarmanna (Gondorf, Germany). On one side of Julia Saturnina's tombstone is a relief depicting a baby covered by firm bandages, perhaps indicating her interests in obstetrics or paediatrics.[14]

One of the impacts of Greek medicine on the Roman world was the employment of public physicians by some communities. Galen reported that, in his day, many cities provided surgeries where doctors could attend the sick.[15] From the distribution of doctors – as attested by inscriptions – across the southern Gallic province of Narbonensis, it seems that most major towns boasted one or more physicians. There is one inscription from Arles, another from Vienne, two from Aix, three from Nimes and seven in Narbonne (the provincial capital).[16]

However, despite all the evidence for physicians across the Empire it is often unclear what led to an individual acquiring the title 'doctor'. There were no examinations, no diplomas, no degrees and no professional licensing procedures in the Roman world. A doctor was simply an individual who claimed the title and carried out treatment for some type of remuneration. Influential contacts, public positions and personal recommendations were much more important than qualifications in enabling doctors to retain patients as well as attracting new clients.[17]

Ulpian, the prominent second century Roman jurist, defined a physician as:

one who promises a cure for any part of the body, or relief from pain, as, for example, an affection of the ear, a fistula, or a toothache; provided he does not employ incantations, imprecations, or exorcisms (to make use of the ordinary term applied to charlatans), for such things as this do not properly belong to the practice of medicine, although there are persons who commend such expedients, and affirm that they have been benefited by them.[18]

The medical training undertaken to become a physician was also extremely variable in terms of time and content. Although some doctors worked as apprentices there was no barrier to others simply setting themselves up in practice with a very minimal level of training.

The physician Galen completed eleven years of study to build the foundations of his career whereas Thessalus of Tralles claimed that the craft of medicine could be learned in six months by anyone.[19]

Starting at the age of seventeen, Galen was a medical student for two years in his native Pergamon before moving to Smyrna. This was followed by five years at Alexandria and a subsequent period of travel within Egypt, furthering his knowledge of pharmacology and anatomy. Alongside his medical training, he also studied philosophy and in his treatise *Quod optimus medicus sit quoque philosophus* (*The Best Doctor Is also a Philosopher*). Galen emphasised the importance of doctors having a solid grounding in logic/reasoning, natural philosophy and ethics.[20]

Returning to Pergamon at the age of twenty-eight, Galen took up his first definitive position as doctor to the town's gladiators, providing him with a wealth of clinical and anatomical experience. Interestingly, according to an epitaph from Aix-en-Provence, the doctor Sextus Julius Felicissimus was attached to the amphitheatre there when he died at the age of nineteen. In addition to '*medicus*', Sextus was given the title of '*alumno*' which probably meant 'pupil'.[21]

In certain cities, and in common with other craftsmen across the Roman world, some physicians formed themselves into medical colleges. At Metz, Sextus Publicius Decamanus was assigned the title '*collegii medicorum liberto*' (freedman of the college of doctors) on his tombstone.[22] Other colleges certainly existed at Turin, Beneventum and Ephesus with evidence of medical contests between members.[23]

During the period of the *Pax Romana,* it was not unusual for physicians to associate themselves with particular schools or sects and follow distinct approaches to caring for their patients. For example, on the memorial stone to the physician Marcus Apronius Eutropus from Vienne in Gaul he was termed '*medico Asclepiadio*' – a follower of Asclepiades of Bithynia. In addition, he was one of the select six Seviri Augustales, appointed for the year by the curia of their city, and chosen according to their wealth and status.[24]

Asclepiades of Bithynia was a Greek physician who developed a new theory of disease, based on the flow of *corpuscles* through *pores* in the body (see Chapter 7). He believed that bodily harmony could be restored by regulating the intake of food and wine, massage, bathing, ambulatory exercise and passive movement involving the use of rocking appliances.[25]

At the time of Galen, the two broad theoretical divisions were between the Empiricist and the Rationalist sects of physicians. However, Galen was probably not unique in basing his practice on both traditions according to the clinical circumstances. The Empiricists attached particular significance to carefully observing patients during the course of an illness, including the response to any treatments. They would also consider any previous findings made by themselves and others in similar situations. A treatment plan would then be selected by comparing the clinical features in their patient with those of conditions that it most resembled. Moreover, if a newly discovered or observed finding contradicted a previously held view, the old idea might be discarded or modified to accommodate the new circumstances.[26]

Empiricist physicians acknowledged that it was useful to try to understand the obvious causes of diseases, but what mattered most was not what caused, but what cured a condition. Celsus, for example, argued that, in the past, effective treatments had been discovered by people wise enough to notice that a specific approach was best to treat a particular condition. He stated that '*the art of medicine was not a discovery following on reasoning, but after the discovery of the remedy, the reason for it was sought out*'.[27] To the Empiricist, it does not matter why a remedy works, only that it does work.

The Rationalists believed in the overriding importance of reason in formulating and adopting a theory concerning the structure and/ or function of the body, and the nature of health and disease. They argued that every medical phenomenon and every disease had a cause (or causes) and that, while many of these were evident, others may be hidden from direct observation. It was then necessary to work out the most appropriate remedies for a disease or disorder linked to the underlying theoretical foundation. The Dogmatics might be considered a sub-division of the Rationalists in that their underlying theory was derived from the Hippocratic focus on the four humours, the four temperaments and the four basic qualities (see Chapter 2). The Pneumatists also had overt Rationalist tendencies but their emphasis was more about *pneuma* in understanding physiology and pathology (see Chapter 2).[28]

Methodism was originally developed from the theories of Asclepiades of Bithynia by the Greek physician Themison. Despite loudly expressed reservations by Galen, it eventually became the dominant medical sect in the late Roman Empire. Methodists argued that all diseases shared some general and plainly visible characteristics, termed commonalities, and that a careful assessment of the patient would provide a good indication of these. According to Themison, there were three major categories of disease, based on 'stricture', 'looseness' or an intermediate, mixed state. To the Methodists, the primary focus of medicine was the specific patient, and phenomena as they were observed in the individual were the only realities of medicine.[29]

Roman medicine and religion were closely intertwined, and many physicians sought divine assistance from a variety of healing deities. For example, dedications by physicians to Aesculapius and Apollo are found widely across the Empire and healing temples often accommodated physicians alongside priests (see Chapter 6). In addition, there were local preferences – for example, according to inscriptions from Ventonimagus in Gaul, the physician Gaius Rufus Eutactus was also closely involved in the cult of Mithras and it has been suggested that he may even have established a health centre near the Mithraeum.[30]

Military medics

Inscriptions bearing the titles of *medicus alae, medicus castrensis/ castrorum, medicus chirurgus, medicus clinicus, medicus cohortis,*

34

medicus duplicarius, *medicus legionis* and *medicus ordinaris* have been found throughout the Roman Empire – in fact, there is currently evidence for medical staff from sixty-seven Roman army sites. Illustrations of treatments of the wounded can also still be clearly seen on a wall painting from Pompeii and on Trajan's column [Plate 5].[31]

There continues to be considerable debate about the precise nature of the Roman army medical service in terms of personnel and organisation. Moreover, it seems likely that, as the Roman army developed and changed over the centuries, so too did the associated health care.[32] It is generally agreed that military medics were appointed by the army, bestowed with a privileged legal position and sanctioned to attend to the soldiers. Their health-related responsibilities would have included ensuring that new recruits were physically fit; providing specialist treatment for battlefield injuries (e.g., wound care and missile extraction), general medical practice and, on some occasions, perhaps advising on healthy locations for the siting of permanent military bases.[33]

Like most frontier provinces, Roman Britain always had a strong military presence and, in addition to the occasional Greek doctor, a range of medical assistance would have been available to the front-line soldiers. At the sharp end were the *capsarii*, the medical orderlies or dressers, the name being derived from the round bandage box (*capsa*) that they carried. These were probably ordinary soldiers concerned mainly with the first aid necessary during battle. Some may have been *immunes* with their medical work being deemed important enough to allow them to be exempted from regular duties. Furthermore, it seems likely that the *capsarii* were under the control of a doctor with the rank of centurion, the *medicus ordinarius*.[34]

A tombstone unearthed from Housesteads reveals the presence of a *medicus ordinarius*. The inscription is translated as: '*To the spirits of the departed (and) to Anicius Ingenuus, medicus ordinarius of the First Cohort of Tungrians: he lived 25 years*' [Plate 6]. The memorial is decorated with the relief of a hare crouching on a plinth under an arched wreath containing a central flower, and each of the upper corners is filled with a carefully carved rosette. Such embellishment is unusual, possibly indicating the status of the individual among his fellow soldiers. The name Ingenuus means freeborn and he may have been the son of a Greek freedman.[35] From Caerleon comes a bronze medical spatula, probably used for applying ointments, inlayed with fine punctate dots indicating the letters: **C. CV............ANILI.** This has been translated as *'the property of CV's (? Cuspius or Curtius) century in charge of Manilianus'*,[36] perhaps with Manilianus being another *medicus ordinarius* [Plate 7].

Whereas Anicius Ingenuus and Manilianus were both middle-ranking soldiers, an inscription from Lyon in memory of a Bononius Gordus refers to him as a *'medicus castrensis'* (camp doctor). Such an individual would have overseen the medical services for the whole fort.[37]

It has been suggested that the more skilled and educated Greek doctors such as Hermogenes and Antiochus (see earlier) may have moved back and forth between civilian and military practice. If this were the case, then they would not have been bound by the usual terms of enlistment for twenty or twenty-five years. Such transitions could also have facilitated the spread of knowledge and practices between the Roman army and local civilian populations. For example, Marcus Ulpius Telesphorus was a medicus in Upper Germany who, according to his memorial inscription, subsequently worked as a civilian doctor.[38]

One of the Vindolanda writing tablets indicates that thirty builders had been required to build a guest-house for Marcus the medicus.[39] Another document refers to the presence of a *valetudinarium* or hospital. As discussed in Chapter 4, there is evidence for *valetudinaria* at several Roman forts and these would have required staffing. The running of such military hospitals was probably delegated to a junior officer: the *optio valetudinarii*.

Eye doctors and oculists

Eye-related issues were a particular concern in the Roman world, perhaps reflecting an ancient view of the eyes as a privileged body part and the transition point between the body and the outside world. For example, Celsus wrote:

> *But there are grave and varied mishaps to which our eyes are exposed; and as these have so large a part both in the service and the amenity of life, they are to be looked after with the greatest care.*[40]

And Pliny the Elder commented:

> *Below the forehead are the eyes, which form the most precious portion of the human body, and which, by the enjoyment of the blessings of sight, distinguish life from death ... In all animals there is no part in the whole body that is a stronger exponent of the feelings, and in man more especially, for it is from the expression of the eye that we detect clemency, moderation, compassion, hatred, love, sadness, and joy. From the eyes, too, the various characters of persons are judged of, according as they are ferocious, menacing, sparkling, sedate, leering, askance, downcast, or languishing. Beyond a doubt it is in the eyes that the mind has its abode: sometimes the look is ardent, sometimes fixed and steady, at other times the eyes are humid, and at others, again, half closed. From these it is that the tears of pity flow, and when we kiss them we seem to be touching the very soul.*[41]

In addition, both Galen and Celsus recommended numerous eye ointments to treat a wide range of eye conditions (see Chapter 5).

Celsus also provided a very clear description of cataract surgery and the eye couching needles to undertake the procedure have been discovered across the Empire, including eight in Gaul[42] (see Chapter 7). From Britain, a military strength report of the First Cohort of Tungrians found at Vindolanda specifically categorises the thirty-one soldiers signed off as unfit into three distinct groups: *aegri* (sick); *volnerati* (wounded); and *lippientes* (eye troubles) [Plate 8].[43]

Votive body parts are linked to religious healing, being donated in hope of a cure or as a thank-you offer, and are widespread across the Roman Empire. From Wroxeter, numerous representations of eyes have come to light – in gold, bronze or carved out of wall plaster [Plate 9].[44] There is evidence for a particular interest in eyes at the temple of Aesculapius at Athens, accounting for 40 per cent of the votive body parts discovered there (see Chapter 6). Eyes votives have also been found at several other healing sanctuaries such as Ponte di Nona (Italy), in addition to at least thirty-six sites in Gaul including Fontes Sequanae, Bû and Les Bollards.[45]

There is some epigraphic evidence for eye doctors (*medicus ocularius*) such as Mantias and Thyrius who might have looked after the Emperor Tiberius [Plate 10].[46] In addition, oculist (or collyrium) stamps are found throughout the Western Roman Empire and, of the 320 recorded to date, over two dozen have been discovered in Britain (see Chapter 5).[47] These were probably used for impressing the name of the maker(s) and the purposes of the treatment onto a hardened block of eye medication (collyrium). The stamps are usually made of greenish schist or steatite and consist of small thin square blocks, generally with an inscription on each of the four edges [Plate 11]. In a few instances, the stone is oblong with two inscribed sides and in one example from Wroxeter, the stamp is circular [Plate 12]. The letters are cut in intaglio form and written from right to left so that when stamped on the collyrium they make an impression that reads from left to right.

Location of find	Name on stamp
Bath	Titus Junianus
Bath	Flavius Litugmus
Biggleswade, Beds	Gaius Valerius Amandus
	Gaius Valerius Valentinus
Caistor-by-Norwich	Publius Anicius Sedatus
Cambridge	Lucius Julius Salutaris
	Marinus
Chester	Quintus Julius Martinus
Cirencester	Minervalis
Cirencester	Atticus
Colchester	Quintus Julius Murranus
Colchester	Lucius Ulpius Deciminus
Colchester	Martialis
Colchester	Publius Claudius Primus
Harrold, Beds	Gaius Junius Tertullus
Kenchester	Titus Vindacius Ariovistus
Kenchester	Aurelius Polychronius
Leicester	Gaius Pal......Gracilis
Littleborough, Notts	Julius Titianus
London	Gaius Silvius Tetricus
Lydney	Julius Jucundus
St Albans	Lucius Julius Ivenis
	Flavius Secundus
Watercrook	Pomponianus Clodianus
Wilcote, Oxon	Maurus
Wroxeter	Tiberius Claudius M.....
Wroxeter	Q.....Lucillianus
York	Julius Alexander

Collyrium stamps from Roman Britain

Whether the British stamps listed in the table (above) represent the names of Romano-British physicians is far from clear. The majority are certainly made of materials easily found in Britain and epigraphic errors as well as the occurrence of typically Celtic names such as Titus Vindacius Ariovistus and Gaius Silvius Tetricus also gives some credence to the essentially local nature of the stamps.

However, across Western Europe over seventy of the names on the stamps have Greek origins and, in one case, the Latin text had simply been transcribed into Greek. In addition, it is uncertain what the exact place of these oculists was in the medical world as none of the stamps identified to date bears the title *medicus*. But some have been found in graves alongside a variety of surgical instruments (scalpels, forceps, hooks, needles and probes) implying that their owners might have been able to undertake some minor surgical procedures too.[48]

It has been suggested that the stamps, rather than the oculists whose names appear on them, travelled the empire and that they may have been handed on from person to person and even down the generations. It has also been proposed that the green colouration of many of the stones might have been considered to confer some sort of magical property to the object. The grave of a doctor at Rheims contained the remains of three stamps. One was blank, the second bore the name Marcellinus and the third was inscribed with the name Gaius Firmius Severus. However, this doctor may not have been either Gaius Severus or Marcellinus.[49] Two of the British stamps bear dual inscriptions and, in relation to the St Albans example, the name Flavius Secundus is executed in a rougher style than that for Lucius Julius Ivenis, perhaps suggesting a succession.

Collyrium stamps are absent from other areas of the Roman Empire and it has been argued that they are a reflection of a different medical system in Gaul, Germany and Britain more appropriate for the requirements of rural communities. Perhaps the sticks of medicament were prepared in bulk at a central location for use by peripatetic eye doctors who made regular circuits round the countryside. This might explain concentrations of stamps from towns and cities such as Colchester, Bavay, Besançon, Amiens, Lyon, Mandeure, Mainz, Rheims and Trier in addition to single finds from numerous rural sites such as the Wilcote villa.[50]

What can the Romans teach us today?
Looking and listening

In the British Museum there is a marble relief of a Greco-Roman doctor from Athens, Jason. The stone carving shows the second-century physician, dressed as a philosopher, seated on a cushioned stool examining an individual with an unnaturally enlarged stomach [Plate 13].[51]

The scene appears relaxed and unhurried with the doctor and the patient looking directly at each other with a sense of mutual trust. Moreover, the medical equipment – in this case a cupping vessel for bloodletting (see Chapter 7) – has been deliberately set to one side of the carving, perhaps indicating its secondary importance in comparison with focusing on the patient.

In *Epidemics* Hippocrates wrote:

The factors which enable us to distinguish between diseases are as follows: First we must consider the nature of man in general and of each individual and the characteristics of each disease. Then we must consider the patient, what food is given to him and who gives it – for this may make it easier for him to take or more difficult – the conditions of climate and locality both in general and in particular, the patient's customs, mode of life, pursuits and age. Then we must consider his speech, his mannerisms, his silences, his habits of sleep or wakefulness and his dreams, their nature and time. Next, we must note how he plucks his hair, scratches or weeps. We must observe his paroxysms, his stools, urine, sputum and vomit. We look for any change in the state of the malady, how often such changes occur and their nature, and the particular changes which induce death or a crisis. Observe, too, sweating, shivering, chill, cough, sneezing, hiccough, the kind of breathing, belching, wind, whether silent or noisy, haemorrhages and haemorrhoids. We must determine the significance of all these signs.[52]

This piece outlines the tremendous importance attached to the detailed observation of patients by classical doctors. Moreover, the assessment did not simply focus on symptoms but also on aspects of a person's behaviour, mental wellbeing, lifestyle and environment. In addition, Hippocrates and Galen both emphasised the requirement to consider how things may have changed over time.[53]

Galen was a particularly astute observer and, in seeking to understand a patient's condition, he also took in a person's surroundings. He was once asked to visit a Sicilian physician who had fallen ill and, as soon as he arrived he picked up a pointer that had not been noticed by others:

just when I entered the house I encountered a person who carried from the bed chamber to the toilet a pan containing a thin bloody serum similar to the watery fluid of freshly slaughtered meat, which is a definite indication of a disease of the liver.[54]

He then went on to describe that:

when I noticed that a little cooking pot, standing at the window, contained a preparation of hyssop in water and honey, I came to the conclusion that this physician believed he suffered from pleurisy, because he had pain in the area of the false ribs as it sometimes occurs during inflammation of the liver.[55]

Sometimes the clues might be more subtle such as those relating to his encounter with a boy suffering from an eating disorder:

Boethus seized me and took me along home to see the boy. People who met us in the street, of whom you were one, also came with

*him. I found that the boy had left the bedroom with his mother to go
to another room where there was a couch on which his mother sat;
a camp bed was attached, a little below the middle of it, on which
she laid the boy, and now she was watching to see that no one came
near him. There was one chair ... and, on the side opposite the
camp bed, by the head of the couch two stools placed together.*[56]

The boy's relocation from his own room, the mother's wariness of
strangers in addition to her physical positioning should lead any doctor –
ancient or modern – to explore other issues in the broader family.

Galen also sought information from third parties:

*I was called in to see a women who was said to lie awake at night,
constantly tossing from one position to another ... I returned the
next day and in a private conversation with the maid on one
subject and another I discovered beyond doubt that she was
racked with grief.*[57]

Aside from observation, listening to patients supplemented with
careful questioning were very important tools for many Roman doctors.
The first-century physician Rufus of Ephesus emphasised that '*the
doctor cannot know*' what he needs to '*by himself*' and that carefully
questioning patients was essential to the acquisition of '*complete and
accurate knowledge*'.[58] He explained that

*You must ask the patient questions. By doing this you will more
accurately recognise anything connected with the sickness, as
well as providing better treatment. Focus on the patient. That
is my first principle: put your enquiries to the patient himself.
From this source you can learn the extent of the person's mental
sickness or health, as well as his physical strength or weakness,
and at the same time the type and location of the sickness he has
been suffering.*[59]

Rufus subsequently went on to list the key areas to focus on that have been summarised by Melinda Letts[60] as:

- Timing of onset
- Whether the complaint is new or recurrent
- The patient's nature and habits and any current divergences from the norm
- Distinguishing between obvious and hidden causes
- The quantity and quality of urine, faeces and saliva compared to dietary intake
- Current patterns of sleep compared to the patient's norm
- Visions and dreams
- Congenital diseases: patterns of recurrence, presentation, previous attacks
- Current dietary and therapeutic regimes, and their effects
- Current food consumption, preferences and reactions
- Pain, especially the distinction of genuine pain from histrionics
- Ease or difficulty of bodily waste processes
- When treating animal bites, whether or not the beast was rabid
- When treating wounds, the type of weapon and wound and the patient's subsequent reactions.

But, as pointed out by Celsus, while questioning patients, doctors must not lose sight of the other key functions of the patient conversation such as gaining an individual's confidence and keeping them calm:

A practitioner of experience does not seize the patient's forearm with his hand, as soon as he comes, but first sits down and with a cheerful countenance asks how the patient finds himself; and if the patient has any fear, he calms him with entertaining talk, and only after that moves his hand to touch the patient.[61]

44

Galen was fascinated by the use of language and did not shy away from harsh criticism of those doctors he thought misunderstood the importance of linguistics. He was particularly keen to ensure that the 'customary use' of a term was clarified as the comprehension of words can vary from person to person, from place to place and from time to time.[62]

He wrote in his treatise on respiration: '*Common words, which then signify no more one thing than the other, confuse and confound the hearer, so that he does not know what is being said until the ambiguity has been distinguished.*'[63] He then went on to point out that language is a joint venture and securing a shared understanding between the parties involved in a clinical conversation is critical.

Galen frequently describes carefully examining patients and he was especially interested in the use of the pulse – writing sixteen books on the topic. Nowadays, we often just count the pulse rate, but he was also concerned with the quality and form of the pulse including '*how the pulse is altered by strivings and fears that suddenly upset the mind*'.[64]

Physical signs of illness can, occasionally, be found in the archaeological record. For example, Romano-Britons with a variety of medical conditions might have visited the healing temple at Lydney Park in Gloucestershire, with some of them drinking the iron-rich waters found there. One person left behind a small votive offering – perhaps in appreciation of a successful cure – in the form of a model forearm. Interestingly the fingernails on the hand are spoon-shaped (termed koilonychia) – a feature that is associated with severe iron deficiency anaemia [Plate 14].[65] Numerous anatomical votives illustrating health conditions such as thyroid disease (goitre), hernias and blindness have also been identified from Gaul.[66] The suggestion that Emperor Maximinus was suffered from acromegaly and gigantism is based on numismatic and literary evidence.[67]

There is little doubt that, compared to our Roman forbears, many modern doctors' observational and listening skills have become blunted. Also, although several studies have continued to emphasise the importance of the information gained by questioning patients, the clinical conversation seems to have been replaced by an increasing range of complex diagnostic equipment. Studies in both the UK and the US have consistently demonstrated that around 80 per cent of diagnoses can be made using the medical history alone with the clinical examination assisting with a further 10 per cent.[68]

Looking back on my own thirty-year career as a general practitioner, I would certainly have benefited from being asked to reflect on the following two statements by Rufus of Ephesus when I was a medical student:

> *One will very often hit the nail on the head by asking the actual patient about events that are unusual for him.*[69]

> *The next thing to ask is whether or not the current problem is among the disorders from which the person commonly suffers, and whether it has happened before. Very often people succumb again to the same things, suffer the same effects and receive the same treatment.*[70]

One issue that seems to be frequently ignored by modern doctors is the communication gap between themselves and many of their patients. No matter whether they correctly and consistently define the patient's presenting symptom, there is still no guarantee that the patient is using the same language or understands technical medical terms and questions. For example, when an individual states that they are dizzy it is important to establish precisely what he or she means.

As pointed out by Galen misunderstandings can also apply to adverbs and adjectives in addition to nouns and verbs. Even if doctors can agree about the terms *productive* cough, *rapid* breathing or *bright-red* bleeding, there is no certainty that patients will share the physician's understanding. The meanings of the words 'often', 'seldom' and 'rarely' can be particularly difficult to pin down.[71]

In addition, doctors vary in their ability to elicit information about symptoms from patients by virtue of, perhaps, differences in the way questions are posed or the way answers are explored. There is always a requirement to ask questions, to clarify comprehension and to interpret responses consistently. As Galen reminds us, nobody wants to appear foolish and it is all-to-easy for patients to say yes/no than indicate poor understanding of the doctor.

Finally, Seneca neatly sums up a patient's perspective on the ideal clinical encounter:

> *If my physician does no more than feel my pulse and class me among those whom he sees in his daily rounds, pointing out what I ought to do or to avoid without any personal interest, then I owe him no more than his fee, because he views me with the eye not of a friend, but of a commander ... Suppose that my physician has spent more consideration upon my case than was professionally necessary; that it was for me, not for his own credit, that he feared: that he was not satisfied with pointing out remedies, but himself applied them, that he sat by my bedside among my anxious friends, and came to see me at the crises of my disorder; that no service was too troublesome or too disgusting for him to perform; that he did not hear my groans unmoved; that among the numbers who called for him I was his favourite case; and that he gave the others only so much time as his care of my health permitted him: I should feel obliged to such a man not as to a physician, but as to a friend.[72]*

Prognosis and prediction
Hippocrates wrote that:

> *it seems to be highly desirable that a physician should pay much attention to prognosis. If he is able to tell his patients when he visits them not only about their past and present symptoms, but also to tell them what is going to happen, as well as to fill in details they have omitted, he will increase his reputation as a*

medical practitioner and people will have no qualms in putting themselves under his care. Moreover, he will be better able to effect a cure if he can foretell, from the present symptoms, the future course of the disease.[73]

For Galen, it was important to '*diagnose the present condition and the prognosis of future, good and bad, that will befall the patient*'.[74] He saw the purpose of prognosis as predicting the likely course of an illness (including the chances of recovery) and to develop a longer-term treatment plan.

In determining an individual's prognosis, he pointed out that it was important to consider any disease or disorder in the context of a particular patient:

The doctor, then, makes a prediction of health or death on no other basis than a precise knowledge of the strength of the disease and the strength of the (patient's) nature ... the resolution of the disease will be quick if the capacity is strong, whereas death will come quickly if the capacity is weak and the disease is stronger.[75]

Nowadays, there is a tendency for doctors to steer away from prognosis focusing much more on diagnosis and treatment. Even when prognosis is considered, the approach is much narrower than in Galen's day, often being restricted to single conditions and outcomes.[76] This change in emphasis in comparison with our ancient forbears might, perhaps, reflect a shift away from an interest in diseased individuals to specific diseases. Also, offering a prognosis feels much less precise with a wider margin of error than suggesting a diagnosis, especially in older adults who might be frail and suffer from a variety of medical problems.[77] And yet many patients are seeking more information from doctors about what the future will bring. In addition, if we don't consider prognosis, there is a risk that some people are offered treatments or operations in which, for them, the potential harms can outweigh any possible benefits.

Interestingly the value of one of Hippocrates' prognostic aphorisms: *'in every disease it is a good sign when the patient's intellect is sound and he enjoys his food; the opposite is a bad sign'*[78] has been examined among a large group of older adults in Manitoba. It was found that poor appetite and poor cognition were linked to increased death rates over a six-year period with particularly poor survival rates if an individual had both features.[79]

Reflecting on the experience of our ancient forbears, it is suggested that we re-consider exploring prognosis in the broader sense as part of any conversation with a patient and their relatives. In addition to a person's age or a specific disease, today's doctors should pay greater attention to treatment goals, comorbidities, cognition and functional status. It is also important to not simply focus on dying but on other outcomes such as discomfort, distress and disability, too, in determining what to do next.[80]

But it will always remain important to keep in mind the imprecise and dynamic nature of prognosis and, as Galen reminds us, prognosis is about developing a longer-term relationship with patients and their families permitting periodic reassessments, reviews and discussions. Galen often warned about the loss of focus on the individual patient and the tendency to over-simplify medical care, making a pertinent analogy with mathematics – there is one level about 'adding up' but a much deeper level concerning 'understanding'.[81]

Regulation and trust

Both the Greeks and the Romans were concerned about the quality and the regulation of doctors. For example, Pliny the Elder wrote that:

The medical profession is the only one in which anybody professing to be a physician is at once trusted, although nowhere else is an untruth more dangerous. We pay however no attention to the danger, so great for each of us is the seductive sweetness of wishful thinking. Besides this, there is no law to punish criminal ignorance, no instance of retribution. Physicians acquire their knowledge from our dangers, making experiments at the cost of our lives. Only a physician can commit homicide with complete impunity.[82]

On their part, some Roman doctors highlighted the importance of professional standards for physicians in addition to other healers. Galen proffered guidance on a doctor's clothes, nails, hair, cleanliness and odour in addition to the appropriate use of technical terms and the correct use of grammar. He also provided patients with a list of questions they should put to a practitioner before engaging them. He particularly recommended observing practitioners at work and noting how well (or badly) they treated the patient – including the accuracy of their prognoses.[83] In selecting the best midwives, the physician and gynaecologist Soranus wrote:

A suitable person will be literate, with her wits about her, possessed of a good memory, loving work, respectable and generally not unduly handicapped as regards her senses, sound of limb, robust, and, according to some people, endowed with long slim fingers and short nails at her fingertips.[84]

The Hippocratic Oath, probably written in the second half of the fifth century BC, constitutes a synopsis of the moral code of ancient Greek medicine (see Appendix 1). The first-century Roman physician Scribonius Largus, in the introduction to his work on pharmacology, quoted from Hippocrates in reminding his readers that '*medicine is that science of healing, not harming*', emphasising that:

All gods and men should hate the doctor whose heart lacks compassion and the spirit of human kindness … Medicine does not measure a man's worth according to his wealth or character,

50

but freely offers its help to all who seek it, and never threatens to harm anyone.[85]

Despite Roman physicians and other healers not being controlled by any formal institutions there was a form of 'social regulation'. Although authority was in the hands of the health care providers, power remained in the hands of patients, with the freedom to choose from within a 'medical marketplace' in determining which therapeutic option to follow. They would also have had the opportunity to attend public displays of medical/anatomical skills, watch processions or medical competitions and gain an insight into a doctor's practice, clientele and reputation. As Galen pointed out, it is much more difficult to bury your mistakes in a small town![86]

Medicine in Rome was often practised in public. The patient might have friends clustering around their bed and the physician may arrive with an entourage or supporters; some even picked up along the way (see the earlier comments concerning Galen's encounter with Boethus). Doctors were also highly competitive, and Galen detailed how he was once ridiculed by Antigenes, the leader of the physicians in his treatment of a patient: *'Look at Eudemus: he is in his sixty third year; he has had three quartan attacks in mid-winter; and Galen promises to cure him.'*

Galen then went on to detail how:

when I correctly declared the basis of the resolution of the second attack, all were astonished; as for the third, they prayed to the gods for my discomfiture. But when that too ended on the day that I had predicted, I gained no slight reputation, not only for my predictions but also for my treatment.[87]

At a broader level, the ruling bodies of some cities and towns offered tax privileges, exemptions from some public obligations or civic salaries to doctors. The Emperor Antoninus Pius set the number of physicians that

51

could be excused from various public duties by a town at between five and ten depending on the population.[88] In addition, the jurist Ulpian wrote that deciding which physicians should be appointed:

> *is the duty of the Order of Decurions and those who possess property therein, in order that, in cases of bodily illness, they may commit themselves and their children to the care of persons selected by themselves, and of whose probity and skill in their profession they are assured.*[89]

Ulpian's statement is also consistent with a reported legal case from Egypt determining whether a local doctor was entitled to claim immunity from liturgies. Interestingly, although the decision hinged on the individual's medical skills, this was something decided by a patient group rather than any medical expert or distant regulatory body. It was not until the creation of the super-elite College of Physicians in Rome in AD 358 that there was any legal reference to the involvement of doctors in the selection of their colleagues.[90]

The social regulation and professional self-regulation within the Roman world have now been replaced by much sturdier fare. Today, in the UK, medical practice is tightly managed by a variety of organisations including the General Medical Council and the Care Quality Commission. Guidelines, protocols, targets and appraisals have also become increasingly important.

The Hippocratic Oath is often viewed as an ancient irrelevance by modern regulators whereas, to others, it remains a powerful representation of the duties and commitments of a physician – doing no harm, acting in the best interests of patients and respecting confidentiality matter as much today as they did in the past.[91]

To many modern doctors, it seems that medical professionalism is being side-lined in favour of instructing doctors to personally collect and assemble data on specific aspects of their care. Subject to a review of such information, doctors are then issued with a 'licence to practise'. In this regard, the second century satirist Lucian made a pertinent observation that will resonate with many of my clinical colleagues: *'Take doctors, for instance: a man of sense, on falling ill, does not send for those who can talk about their profession best, but for those who have trained themselves to accomplish something in it.'*[92] Also, although very few modern doctors have their clinical care directly observed (as was the case in Galen's day) patients are now assured that robust systems are in place to judge a doctor's honesty, competence and reliability.

Defensive medical practice is defined as giving treatment or undertaking tests or procedures for the purpose of protecting the doctor from criticism rather than diagnosing or treating a patient. My own research has demonstrated a significant escalation in such practice that can be correlated with the increased regulatory burden.[93] How does this trend square with the statement in the Hippocratic Oath *'I will use treatment to help the sick according to my ability and judgement, but never with a view to injury or wrongdoing'* (see Appendix 1)?

At all times and in all places there will always be healers who are 'bad apples' but striving for a perfect regulatory system for physicians is both futile and foolhardy. Dishonest doctors will always play the system and there is a risk that, over time, a 'licence to practise' simply becomes a 'licence to deceive'.[94] Also, not everything that counts can be counted such as the basic humanity that shines through the writings of Scribonius Largus, Galen and Celsus. Some modern medical philosophers and ethicists have suggested that the work of Scribonius Largus could even form the basis for a new approach to rebuilding medical morality.[95] There is clearly much we can learn from our Roman forbears about the best way for patients to be able to place their trust intelligently in doctors and other healers.

CHAPTER 4

Architecture and Health

Rome is often credited with improving public health by encouraging the building of aqueducts and bathhouses, in addition to developing efficient waste disposal arrangements. The first hospitals were also established by the Roman army and several Greek healing sanctuaries underwent structural modifications during the imperial period with a greater emphasis on secular and holistic care (see Chapter 6).

But some of Rome's construction projects might have had detrimental effects on the wellbeing of the population. For example, the advent of excellent roads and improved communications would have contributed to the ease with which diseases were spread. Within Britain, the increased contacts with other areas of the Empire following the invasion of AD 43, combined with a gradual trend to greater urbanisation, led to both the introduction and the spread of new diseases. There is palaeopathological evidence for population-density dependent illnesses such as tuberculosis and leprosy first occurring in Britain during the Roman period. Moreover, according to Roberts and Cox, the prevalence of non-specific infections identified from excavated skeletal remains rises from 1.5 per cent in the Iron Age to 6.7 per cent under the Romans.[1]

The second century Antonine Plague, probably smallpox, and a by-product of the Parthian War in the East, rapidly spread to Italy.[2] The historian Dio Cassius, who was a young man at the time, wrote: *'A pestilence occurred, the greatest of any of which I have knowledge; for two thousand persons often died in Rome in a single day.'*[3]

Subsequently, river traffic along the Rhine and Rhone was particularly important in moving the disease closer to the English Channel and into the new Roman ports that had been built at Gloucester and London.[4] It has even been suggested that it reached Hadrian's Wall based on the finding of an inscription at Housesteads translated '*to the gods and goddesses according to the interpretation of the oracle of the Clarian Apollo*'. A dozen similar dedications have been found scattered across the Empire and they are considered to represent a centralised anti-plague initiative.[5]

Fifteen years ago, the remains of at least ninety-one hurriedly buried individuals were uncovered in a mass grave in Gloucester. The pit contained a tangle of skeletal parts, so contorted and intermeshed as to imply that all the bodies had been tipped in at the same time. Although it is impossible to prove that the individuals died due to smallpox – as this would often kill people and leave no signs on the surviving skeletal remains – the dating evidence from the grave is in keeping with burial at the time of the Antonine Plague. Moreover, alternative explanations for a mass grave of this type – warfare or poverty – are not consistent with the osteological findings. Nearly half of the individuals were young adults with no signs of malnutrition, injuries, or chronic illnesses.[6]

Although we often associate the Romans with farms and urban development, it is important to appreciate that, even in later Roman Britain, only about 1 per cent of the rural population inhabited villas and 6.5 per cent lived in towns.[7] Many people in rural areas continued to occupy round houses along similar lines to their Iron Age ancestors. These individuals would have been exposed to indoor pollution as a result of co-habitation with animals and cooking, in addition to various cottage industries. In the towns the situation might have been particularly difficult for the poor with their homes serving as workshops as well as living quarters.

In considering the interaction between classical architecture and health there is a risk of viewing structures such as aqueducts or bathhouses solely through modern eyes. For example, even today, the termination of the long-defunct Dorchester Roman aqueduct is marked with an impressively reconstructed fountain reminding visitors of the engineering achievements of their Roman forbears [Plate 15]. By the imperial period, aqueducts had come to be regarded as one of the essential features of fully developed civilised urban life, and it might even be suggested that their existence says more about the aspirations of a provincial town to appear 'Roman' than any particular concern for public health. The over-riding imperative for Roman towns to construct aqueducts is clearly illustrated by a letter from Pliny the Younger to the Emperor Trajan concerning the town of Nicomedia (Turkey):

> *The citizens of Nicomedia, Sir, have spent 3,318,000 sesterces on an aqueduct which they abandoned before it was finished and finally demolished. Then they made a grant of 200,000 sesterces towards another one, but this too was abandoned.*[8]

Bathhouses can also be viewed as an expression of Roman power and the adoption of Roman civilisation rather than simply about washing. In his biography of Agricola, Tacitus wrote:

> *The following winter was spent on schemes of social betterment. Agricola had to deal with people living in isolation and ignorance, and therefore prone to fight; and his object was to accustom them to a life of peace and quiet by the provision of amenities. He therefore gave private encouragement and official assistance to the building of temples, public squares, and good houses … And so the population was gradually led into the demoralising temptations of arcades, baths, and sumptuous banquets. The unsuspecting Britons spoke of such novelties as 'civilization', when in fact they were only a feature of their enslavement.*[9]

Water supply and sewers

Sextus Julius Frontinus, having already served as a governor of Britain, was appointed *curator aquarum* (supervisor of the aqueducts) by the

Emperor Nerva in AD 97. In *De aquis urbis Romae* (*The Aqueducts of Rome*), he presented a description of the water-supply of Rome, including the laws relating to its use and maintenance.[10] He also provided information on the history, sizes and discharge rates of all the nine aqueducts of Rome at the time he was writing. Most drew their supply from a river or a spring rather than a reservoir and, for example, Frontinus explained how the water from the healing springs of Camenae was now brought directly into Rome by such structures.

The most common reason to construct an aqueduct was to feed the public baths but the water might also have been used for fountains, flushing drains or distributed to private households. On occasion, they served to support mining operations, drove water wheels for mills and irrigated farms or gardens. Today, the archaeological remains of numerous Roman stone aqueducts can still be found spread across the area occupied by the Empire and, in Gaul alone, there is evidence for at least three hundred.[11]

Water flowed along aqueducts through conduits due to a slight overall downward gradient. All the systems identified to date functioned based on a constant gravitational flow and, except for maintenance or repair works, the supply was never shut off completely. If necessary, any excess water could be diverted to another branch or be used to flush the sewers. Water conservation was not a major issue for the Romans or a priority for Roman engineers!

Most conduits were buried beneath the ground and followed the contours of the terrain; obstructing peaks were circumvented or, less often, tunnelled through. Bridges and viaducts, sometimes very large, might be needed to cross intervening valleys. For cities built on hills and surrounded by plains, there was often an additional requirement for the final section to be supported by a series of arcades to maintain the water level and to regulate the flow rate.[12]

Another mechanism to take water across a valley was by means of an inverted siphon. At Lyon, water flowed into a large header tank and down into the valley within nine thickened lead pipes. Hydrostatic pressure would then force the water back up the other side to a receiving tank set at a slightly lower level than the header tank. If the gully was particularly deep, the pipes were sometimes taken across the bottom on a slightly raised bridge (venter), probably to alleviate the enormous internal pressures at the base of the siphons.[13]

Many aqueduct systems included settling tanks, which would have helped to remove water-borne debris or sediment. Calcium carbonate encrustation (sinter) along the sides of the channel also had to be chipped off manually as it could dramatically restrict water flow.[14] On arrival at the city, the water would pour into a large distribution tank (*castellum*) from which supplies branched off to other parts of the city carried by open conduits or within pipes.

Although Roman Britain cannot boast an equivalent of structures such as the Pont du Gard in Gaul, evidence for aqueducts and water distribution systems can still be found at sites of forts, *coloniae, civitas* capitals and many smaller Romano-British towns.[15]

At Lincoln (*Lindum Colonia*), the aqueduct consisted of a series of interlocking earthenware pipes, each nearly a metre long and with a maximum internal diameter of 14cm. The whole pipeline was also encased in a waterproof concrete jacket approximately 38cm in cross section [Plate 16]. The Lincoln aqueduct has been a source of interest and some controversy for many years and even the origin of the water supply remains an area of debate. It was once considered that the water was drawn from the Roaring Meg spring just north of Lincoln but this is 20 metres lower than the upper city of *Lindum* and a system to raise the water to feed into the aqueduct would have been required. An alternative suggestion is that the water was tapped from springs on the higher ground further north, with the aqueduct crossing over the dip adjacent to the Roaring Meg spring by means of a bridge structure. Hydrostatic pressure would then have driven the water across the bridge and up into the city (using the inverted siphon system as at Lyon) with the encased pipe having to withstand considerable internal pressures.[16]

The *civitas* capitals at Leicester, Dorchester and Wroxeter were supplied by leats rather than pipes.[17] The Dorchester example followed the contours to the north-west of the town, running for over 15km at a gentle gradient of 1 in 1750 [Plates 17 and 18]. There were probably three channels and, although only one ever worked, it seems likely that the aqueduct could have supplied the requirements of the town.[18]

One of the outstanding questions about aqueducts in the context of Roman Britain is why were they constructed anyway? There was certainly no shortage of water in Roman Britain, and in London, for example, the fifty wells identified to date, in addition to the many natural springs, could easily have supplied all the city's drinking water requirements.[19] Even at Lincoln a massive well sunk right through the limestone layers and into the lias clay at the site of the Roman forum would have served as a major source of water for the upper city.[20]

Contemporary literary evidence concerning Roman sewers and latrines is extremely meagre. However, visiting Chester a thousand years after the departure of the Romans, the monk Ranulf Higden wrote admiringly: '*There be ways under the ground vaulted marvellously with stonework, chambers having arched roofs overhead, huge stones engraved with the names of ancient men.*'[21] Even today, the sewage system in York can be followed for 44 metres and there is evidence for side channels, manhole covers and sluices.[22]

At Housesteads Fort the Roman latrines can still be clearly identified [Plate 19]. The visible remains consist of a deep sewer flowing around a central platform and the sewer pit would have been spanned by a continuous row of wooden lavatory seats. The small central water channel provided water for washing and it has been suggested that, in northern Britain, moss was used as a form of lavatory paper.[23] Alternative options to clean the buttocks after toileting included a sponge fixed to a stick (*tersorium*) or circular fragments of ceramic (*pessoi*).[24]

Both single (*latrinae*) and multi-seater (*foricae*) toilets are found at many Roman sites and there were probably between 200 and 300 in Pompeii. Some of these domestic toilets would have been supplied with piped water, which might have assisted in washing away waste, aided by sloping tiled floors. There is also evidence that the waste-water from the bathhouse in the House of the Faun was used to flush the associated latrine.[25]

Frontinus commented on the use of overflow water from aqueduct reservoirs to wash through the sewers in Rome[26] and, at Wroxeter, the water from the open channel aqueduct probably served a similar purpose.[27] At Housesteads, the location of the latrines at the lower south-east corner of the fort would have permitted surface water to be channelled to cleanse the associated sewer.[28]

Bathhouses and spas

A visit to the baths was one of the great pleasures for the Romans and many individuals would have attended every day. Bathhouses varied from imperial *thermae* to municipal *balaneae*, in addition to numerous smaller private concerns.

The *thermae* are generally distinguished from the *balaneae* by their size, lofty magnificence and luxury with marble, mosaics, frescoes, paintings and statues. Entering would have been a sensory adventure with visitors being subjected to novel sights, sounds (including echoes), smells and various new tactile experiences as they walked around.[29]

Bathhouses were extremely widespread across the empire and, by the fourth century AD, it is estimated that there were 856 baths plus 10 *thermae* within Rome. Even the smaller town of Timgad in Algeria, with a population of around 6,000, boasted seven bathhouses.[30] In relation to the port of Smyrna, the orator and author Aelius Aristides lamented that '*it had so many baths that you would be at a loss to know where to bathe*'.[31]

Although nowadays we might view the function of a bathhouse as a cleansing establishment, the Romans might have used it for many other purposes including commerce, socialising, cosmetic procedures, eating and drinking, exercise, entertainment, and for various medical and physical treatments (see Chapter 7). Many larger bathing establishments – particularly the *thermae* – occasionally included lecture halls, libraries, shrines, art galleries, small shops, galleries and theatrical stages. Some also accommodated performances by actors, musicians, jugglers and acrobats.[32]

An inscription from Moesia stating that the villagers of Petra *'contributed to the building of the bath for the sake of their bodily health'*[33] emphasises the perceived link between bathing and wellbeing. Statues of the healing deities Aesculapius and Hygieia were also particularly common at bathhouses and some physicians as well as medical masseurs would have offered their services within such establishments. There is suggestive evidence for some minor surgical procedures being undertaken at bathhouses based on finds of medical instruments at Xantan, Pompeii and Caerleon.[34] The drain from the Weissenburg baths produced an inlaid silver scalpel, in addition to a possible medical spoon, probes and tweezers. Five teeth recovered from the drains at Caerleon – two of which showed some evidence of decay – implies that dental extractions might have been performed there.[35] Celsus[36] indicated that baths had a role in treating eye problems, and collyrium stamps (see Chapters 3 and 5) have been discovered associated with the baths at Trier, in addition to a possible slate medicine grinding palate and glass stirring rod from Caerleon.[37]

Gentle activity prior to bathing was a key part of the bathing process and Pliny the Younger described the preparatory steps before entering the baths in his letter to Fuscus Salinator: *'... then I have another walk, am oiled, take exercise and have a bath'*.[38] Ball games were a frequent pursuit as suggested by Galen in *'De parvae pilae exertio'* (*On Exercise with a Small Ball*)[39] and Martial listed four varieties: *pila paganica* (feather-ball), *follis* (bladder-ball), *harpastum* (scrimmage-ball) and *pila trigonalis* (a game with three players trying to catch the ball).[40] In some places there were colonnaded courtyards for exercising (*palaestra or gymnasia*) associated with the baths, and even athletic competitions.

Undoubtedly, public baths were busy places but all the activity going on was clearly an issue for Seneca:

Picture me with a babel of noise going on all about me, staying right over the public bathhouse. ... When the strenuous types are doing their exercises, swinging weight-laden hands about, I hear the grunting as they toil away – or go through the motions of toiling away – at them, and the hissings and strident gasps every time they expel their pent up breath. When my attention turns to a less active fellow who is contenting himself with an ordinary inexpensive massage, I hear the smack of a hand pummelling his shoulders, the sound varying according as it comes down flat or cupped. But if on top of this some ball player comes along and starts shouting out the score, one's done for! Now add someone starting up a brawl, and someone else caught thieving, and the fellow who likes the sound of his voice in the bath, and the people who leap into the pool with a tremendous splash. Going beyond those sounds which are straightforward if nothing else, call to mind the hair remover, repeatedly giving vent to his shrill and penetrating cry the better to advertise his presence, never silent unless it be while he is plucking someone's armpits and making the client yell for him! Then think of the various cries of the man selling drinks, and the one selling sausages and the other selling pastries, and all the ones hawking for the catering shops, each publicising his wares with a distinctive cry of his own.[41]

Although the precise layouts of bathhouses varied they usually contained three principal chambers graduated in temperature: a cold room (*frigidarium*), a warm room (*tepidarium*) [Plate 20] and a hot room (*caldarium*). In general, the bathing sequence went from warm to hot being terminated by a period within the *frigidarium*. In the *frigidarium*, bathers could cool down slowly or, in some cases, sit in a cold bath, have cold water poured water over them, or swim in a cold pool (*natatio*). The *caldarium* was generally equipped with a hot bath in which individuals bathed after having been oiled and scraped down with a strigil. In some bathhouses there were even specific sweating rooms – *laconicum* (dry heat) or *sudatorium* (steamy, wet heat) as well as dedicated locations for massaging with warm oils (*uncturarium*) or scraping down (*destrictarium*).[42]

Spas are bathing establishments that were specifically patronised because of the perceived medicinal qualities of the water such as its temperature and/or its mineral content (see Chapter 7) [Plate 21]. Many subsequently developed into towns incorporating the name *Aquae* such as *Aquae Sulis* (Bath), *Aquae Granni* (Aachen), *Aquae Sextiae* (Aix-en-Provence) or *Aquae Helveticae* (Baden, Switzerland).[43] Tacitus referred to the latter as a place that '*had been built up into the semblance of a town and was much resorted to for its beauty and healthful waters*'.[44]

The springs around Baiae were especially popular, being recommended by medical authors such as Celsus.[45] Over the years, several bulbous glass flasks have come to light that are etched with scenes from Baiae and neighbouring Puteoli. These objects might have been tourist souvenirs or religious objects and they show the key architectural elements of the sites. Many of the images are labelled and the buildings illustrated include theatres, amphitheatres, temples, baths, sun terraces and palestrae.[46] A silver bowl from Otanes near Castro Urdiales in Spain details scenes showing the various activities at a spa: collecting water, drinking, making offerings and even transporting water away by cart.[47]

In many spas there would have been an overlap between secular and divine healing (see Chapter 6). At the Badenweiler spa (*Aquae Villae*) several medical instruments including a bronze urinary catheter have been discovered alongside statues of Mercury and votive offerings.[48] Collyrium eye stamps have been found associated with the spas at Bath (*Aquae Sulis*), Néris-les-Bains (*Aquae Nerii*) and Vichy (*Aquae Calidae*).[49]

Spas might also have provided places where sick or wounded soldiers could have recuperated and rehabilitated. A third of the Roman visitors mentioned on inscriptions found at Bath were military, including two centurions, a number of legionaries and a Spanish cavalryman.[50] Lucius Latinius Macer, a native of Verona and praefectus castrorum of the Legio IX Hispana in the early second century AD dedicated an altar to Apollo at Aachen.[51] But a petition submitted by the residents of a Thracian village to the Emperor Gordian suggests that some soldiers visiting the nearby health spa might have been overstepping the mark in demanding free food from the locals.[52]

Although bathing was seen as offering health benefits, it was not free of dangers. There is evidence for occasional drownings and some Romans even worried about 'bath demons' with protective symbols and amulets being found in several bathhouses. Also, not all establishments were magnificent structures; some being dirty, decrepit and in danger of collapse.[53]

The Romans didn't use thermometers so the temperatures of *caldaria* might have varied significantly. Seneca raised concerns about:

> *the kind of heat that has recently come into fashion, more like that of a furnace – so much so indeed that a slave convicted in a criminal charge might well be sentenced to being bathed alive! There doesn't seem to be any difference now between 'your bath's warm' and 'your bath's boiling'.*[54]

Perhaps as a result of having had his knee badly burnt on being carried into the baths, Fronto expressed a preference for natural springs:

> *to me the steaming grottoes of Baiae are better than your bath-furnaces, in which the fire is kindled with cost and smoke, and anon goes out. But the natural heat of the former is at once pure and perpetual, as grateful as it is gratuitous.*[55]

It seems likely that other visitors would also have been affected by the fumes, smoke and gases from the combustion (or partial combustion) of carbon-based fuels.

There were probably infection risks associated with bathing, especially if the water was changed infrequently. Marcus Aurelius wrote: *'What do the baths bring to your mind? Oil, sweat, dirt, greasy water, and everything that is disgusting'*[56] and Pliny the Elder commented that individuals were more likely to pick up various parasitic insects from visiting public baths.[57] Also, although Celsus was a great advocate of the health benefits of bathing (see Chapter 7), he specifically stated that it should be avoided for individuals with wounds *'for this makes the wound both wet and dirty, and then there is a tendency for gangrene to occur'*.[58] There can be little doubt that treating those with certain illnesses in crowded bathhouses would also have contributed to the spread of infectious diseases. Hadrian's measure to give the sick exclusive use of the baths until the eighth hour was, perhaps, motivated by a wish to protect the healthy from the unhealthy.[59] In some spas – for example at *Aquae Segetae* (Sceaux-du-Gâtinais) – there might have been two thermal baths … one for the public and another for individuals seeking cures.[60]

A mosaic from the Sabratha baths showing three strigils, two bath clogs, and one oil flask is inscribed *'Salvom Lavisse'*, translated as *'to bathe is healthy'*, but it has also been interpreted as a cryptic warning *'to bathe safely'*. Likewise, at Timgad baths the words *'Bene Lava'* might suggest having a pleasant as well as a safe bath.[61]

However, perhaps the final word on the Roman view of bathing is best provided by an epitaph on the tomb of Tiberius Claudius Secundus: *'Baths, wine, and sex corrupt our bodies, but baths, wine, and sex make life worth living.'*[62]

Hospitals (*Valetudinaria*)

Although Roman army hospitals certainly existed, their presence at many military sites is contentious. There are certainly epigraphic references to *valetudinaria* (e.g. at Stojnik and Vindolanda) in addition to the individuals in charge of such hospitals – *optio valetudinarii* (e.g. at Lambiensis and Bonn).[63] In *De munitionibus castrorum* (*Fortifying a Roman Camp*), Hyginus wrote about the careful siting of the *valetudinarium* within the fort, well away from the *fabrica* and *veterinarium*, allowing the patients peace and quiet.[64]

The first *valetudinarium* to be recognised by archaeologists was found at Neuss (*Novaesium*) in 1904. This identification was based on its design, location in the fort and the finding of possible medical instruments within the building – ten probes and four scalpels. Some seeds of henbane as well as carbonised centaury were also discovered. These might have been used by the Romans as sedatives and for wound healing.[65]

At Housesteads, a possible hospital has been identified behind the *principia* away from the general hustle and bustle of the fort [Plates 22 and 23]. In common with the exemplar at Neuss, it has a rectangular footprint with a series of small rooms arranged around a central courtyard. It also seems that there was a possible ambulatory around the inside of the building surrounded by a low wall that supported a colonnade. In addition, it had its own latrine in the south-west corner and cooking hearths. Although no surgical instruments have been unearthed at the hospital site, a spoon-scoop has been discovered that could have been used to remove ointments and powders from wide-necked jars and bottles. Elsewhere in the fort, ear probes, an ointment palate, a spoon-probe and a sharp hook (used for seizing and holding the margins of wounds) have come to light as well as the tombstone of the *medicus ordinarius* Anicius Ingenuus (see Chapter 3).[66]

It has been estimated that *valetudinaria* were designed for acute injuries or illnesses being only able to accommodate up to 5 per cent of a unit.[67] As suggested earlier, soldiers requiring long-term care or convalescence might have been granted sick leave to recuperate elsewhere. Hopeless or terminal cases may have been sent away too;

both Gaius Modestus from the second legion and Julius Vitalis an armorer of the twentieth legion died at Bath in their twenties.[68]

There might also have been some civilian hospitals and sick bays for slaves at large country estates. However, in general most care was undertaken in people's homes as indicated by Tacitus in his report of the collapse of an amphitheatre at Fidenae:

Immediately after the catastrophe, leading Romans threw open their homes, providing medical attention and supplies all round. In those days Rome, for all its miseries, recalled the practice of our ancestors, who after great battles had lavished gifts and attention on the wounded.[69]

What can the Romans teach us today?

Public health is about disease prevention and health protection in addition to the promotion of better health;[70] architecture can have impacts on all these aspects of population health. Although the Roman theories and understanding of health and disease are distinct from ours, they clearly did appreciate the importance of safe and reliable water supplies. Also, they generally disposed of their dead outside the city boundaries[71] and their attempts at draining marshes might have done something to reduce the incidence of malaria.[72]

However, in comparison with our modern biomedical perspective, it is suggested that humoral theory (see Chapter 2) encouraged a much greater focus on the broader determinants of health. This included the potential impacts of the environment (including buildings and landscape) on an individual's wellbeing.

Health protection

Protecting health is about the identification, prevention and mitigation of the impacts of various threats to the public health.[73] In *De aquis urbis Romae*, Frontinus highlighted the importance that the Romans attached to the availability of running water. He emphasised that, as *curator aquarum*, his responsibilities were about '*the convenience but also the health and even the safety of the City*'.[74] But whether he had adopted a similar perspective during his time as governor of Britain is difficult to gauge. Certainly, many of the 'aqueducts' from Roman Britain were little more than lined channels or single pipelines and it has been argued that few of them could have provided much water for domestic consumption. For example, the 'aqueduct' supplying the fort at Brough-on-Noe probably delivered about as much water as an average domestic tap does today.[75] Furthermore, although many forts possessed aqueduct supplies, perhaps because of the ready availability of skilled military personnel such as surveyors and architects, some of this water may have been used for purposes other than human consumption.[76]

Although the Lincoln aqueduct was one of the most impressive and technologically sophisticated of the Roman civic water supply systems in Britain, doubts continue to be expressed about whether it actually worked, or even flowed in the right direction! If the source of the water was from the limestone ridge in the Lincolnshire Wolds, it seems surprising that no limescale deposits have yet been found in any of the pipes excavated.[77] The Dorchester aqueduct tapped the sluggish river Frome, and the quality or safety of the water can hardly have been improved by its long journey within an open leat.[78]

Many of the sewage systems within Roman Britain were certainly not as impressive as those found at, for example, York, Chester or Lincoln.[79] Cirencester just had a timber-lined gully running down the middle of the street and some drains only extended a short way beyond the walls – perhaps just sufficient to remove foul smells – before discharging into the town ditch.[80] Cesspits for waste – often located near kitchens – were a much more common arrangement.[81] The situation in Britain was probably replicated in many other provinces and, in relation to the port of Smyrna, Strabo the Greek geographer wrote:

> *But there is one error, not a small one, in the work of the engineers, that when they paved the streets they did not give them underground drainage; instead, filth covers the surface, and particularly during rains, when the cast-off filth is discharged upon the streets.*[82]

Based on a review of the available evidence from latrines, burials and coprolites (preserved faeces) it is suggested that intestinal parasites such as whipworm, roundworm and amoeba were quite prevalent during the Roman period, in addition to fleas, lice and fish tapeworm. Mitchell argues that this demonstrates that the availability of facilities such as latrines, aqueducts or bathhouses had little impact on infectious diseases.[83] However, in contrast to these findings, a detailed examination of the bioarchaeological remains from the four *coloniae* at York, Chester, Gloucester and Colchester concluded that they had been kept reasonably clean.[84]

Aside from infectious diseases, concerns have also been raised about the potential health impacts of the use of lead piping in water systems [Plate 24]. Moreover, recent work has revealed that some excavated Roman bones from London contain seventy times more lead than is the case for pre-Roman Iron Age examples.[85] These findings echo others demonstrating increased lead levels within dental enamel.[86]

For children, lead poisoning can cause learning difficulties, behavioural problems, stunted growth, anaemia and kidney damage. In adults, the consequences range from infertility to muscle, nerve and joint disorders. However, it is important to be aware that there were many other sources of lead in Roman Britain including from cooking vessels, imported wine, cosmetics and even some medical treatments.[87]

In the early Republic, the Romans had discovered the mechanism of sweetening and preserving sour wines with lead-containing additives. They found that *sapa*, a syrup prepared by concentrating must in a lead vessel, kept wine from spoiling and gave it an agreeable flavour. Based on Roman descriptions for preserving wine in this fashion, Eisinger repeated the process and found that the ingestion of such lead-preserved wine would provide an individual with a dose of 20mg of lead per litre of wine drunk.[88] The chronic toxicity limit above which symptoms of lead poisoning will occur is one fortieth of this.

But, irrespective of the exact contribution of lead piping to any lead toxicity among the Romans, it is important to be aware that the Roman architect Vitruvius was aware of the potential problem and even suggested a solution:

Water-supply by earthenware pipes has these advantages. First, if any fault occurs in the work, anybody can repair it. Again, water is much more wholesome from earthenware pipes than from lead pipes. For it seems to be made injurious by lead, because white lead is produced by it; and this is said to be harmful to the human body.[89]

An overall view on the adequacy of health protection arrangements under the Romans is provided by Scobie who argues that, in comparison with modern Western industrial societies, the Roman world falls short. Aside from the issues highlighted above concerning the adequacy of the drains and water supply systems in the provinces, it is suggested that, even within Rome, large numbers of inhabitants lived in unsafe and unsanitary conditions. There would also have been an enormous gulf separating the rich from the poor with respect to access to medical care, waste disposal and decent housing. Huts were often erected against public buildings or in porticos and some people had to find refuge in tombs, under stairs or in cellars.[90] Scobie concludes that

70

Baudel's description of Paris in the sixteenth and seventeenth centuries might equally well be applied to ancient Rome:

> *chamber pots ... continued to be emptied out of windows; the streets were sewers. For a long time, Parisians relieved themselves under a row of yews in the Tuileries; driven from here by the Swiss guards, they betook themselves to the banks of the Seine, which was equally revolting to eye and nose.*[91]

However, the Romans did achieve a remarkable degree of standardisation in the provision of certain basic facilities. For example, across the major towns of Britain there is archaeological evidence for functioning aqueducts and sewers at a dozen sites but a triumphal arch at only one (St Albans).[92] And, as pointed out by Frontinus: '*With such an array of indispensable structures carrying so many waters, compare, if you will, the idle Pyramids or the useless, though famous, works of the Greeks.*'[93]

In relation to both their predecessors and their successors, the Roman approach would certainly have contributed to some improvements in the public health. Even today it is worth reflecting that at least 2 billion people use a drinking water source contaminated with faeces[94] and a similar number do not have basic sanitation facilities such as toilets or latrines.[95] In addition, the absolute number of people living in slums or informal settlements has now grown to over one billion and this is likely to rise further with increasing urbanisation.[96]

Enhancing wellbeing

In considering the role of architecture in protecting health Vitruvius commented on the importance of selecting healthy sites for building new settlements:

> *Now this will be high and free from clouds and hoar frost, with an aspect neither hot nor cold but temperate. Besides, in this*

way a marshy neighbourhood shall be avoided. For when the morning breezes come with the rising sun to a town, and clouds rising from these shall be conjoined, and, with their blast, shall sprinkle on the bodies of the inhabitants the poisoned breaths of marsh animals, they will make the site pestilential.[97]

And he even suggested a diagnostic test for assessing the suitability of a site:

... I vote for the revival of the old method. For the ancients sacrificed the beasts which were feeding in those places where towns or fixed camps were being placed and they used to inspect the livers.[98]

But Vitruvius was also concerned with the role of buildings in enhancing wellbeing. He wrote that:

the open spaces which are between the colonnades under the open sky, are to be arranged with green plots; because walks in the open are very healthy, first for the eyes, because from the green plantations, the air being subtle and rarefied.[99]

In accordance with the humoral theory, the Romans attached particular significance to the impact of pure air, movement, sleep and diet on physical and mental wellbeing (see Chapter 2). In terms of architecture there are frequent references to considering the importance of light, air, space, setting, sights and sounds,[100] in addition to locating and designing structures to encourage movement (also see Chapters 2 and 6).

Many bathhouses, especially the thermae, were renowned for their physical beauty with an emphasis on light, décor and space. Clearly, bathhouses were not just about bathing and the health benefits from taking the waters might have been magnified by the uplifting environment and the positive social interactions with other members of the community. Fagan points out that the size of the specific 'bathing' areas within bathhouses reduced over the course of the early empire from 33 per cent in the forum baths at Pompeii to 18 per cent in the Baths of Trajan.[101]

The satirist Lucian wrote about the Baths of Hippias designed, he stated, by an architect who was '*a leader in harmony and music as well as in engineering and geometry*':

The entrance is high, with a flight of broad steps of which the tread is greater than the pitch, to make them easy to ascend. On entering, one is received into a public hall of good size, with ample accommodations for servants and attendants. On the left are the lounging rooms, also of just the right sort for a bath, attractive, brightly lighted retreats. Then, beside them, a hall, larger than need be for the purposes of a bath, but necessary for the reception of the rich. Next, capacious locker-rooms to undress in, on each side, with a very high and brilliantly lighted hall between them, in which are three swimming-pools of cold water; it is finished in Laconian marble, and has two statues of white marble in the ancient technique, one of Hygieia, the other of Aesculapius.

On leaving this hall, you come into another which is slightly warmed instead of meeting you at once with fierce heat; it is oblong, and has a recess at each side. Next it, on the right, is a very bright hall, nicely fitted up for massage, which has on each side an entrance decorated with Phrygian marble, and receives those who come in from the exercising-floor. Then near this is another hall, the most beautiful in the world, in which one can sit or stand with comfort, linger without danger and stroll about with profit. It also is refulgent with Phrygian marble clear to the roof. Next comes the hot corridor, faced with Numidian marble. The hall beyond it is very beautiful, full of abundant light and aglow with colour like that of purple hangings. It contains three hot tubs.

When you have bathed, you need not go back through the same rooms, but can go directly to the cold room through a slightly warmed apartment. Everywhere there is copious illumination and full indoor daylight. Furthermore, the height of each room is just, and the breadth proportionate to the length; and everywhere great beauty and loveliness prevail.[102]

Of particular note are the five distinct references to light and the focus on visual beauty. In recent years, we have begun to learn more about the significant mental health benefits derived from natural light.[103] There is also evidence that artwork can be effective in soothing stress and providing distraction from pain, especially when it depicts nature.[104]

Nowadays – and for good reason – we have a much greater focus on hospital-based care than was the case in the Roman world. But, as pointed out by Celsus hospital care does have its downsides:

those who treat cattle and horses, since it is impossible to learn from dumb animals particulars of their complaints, depend only upon common characteristics … Again, those who take charge of large valetudinaria, because they cannot pay full attention to individuals, resort to these common characteristics.[105]

Certainly, some of my patients could benefit enormously from their care being less focused on visiting hospitals; instead, being looked after and monitored at home.[106] Also, for those who do require in-patient services, more thought needs to be given to how the design of hospital buildings impacts on a person's wellbeing. A study from 1984 found that surgical patients assigned to rooms with windows looking out on a natural scene recovered more quickly and required fewer pain killers than individuals in similar rooms with windows facing a brick wall.[107]

Also, the growing evidence that higher daylight exposure reduces pain, underscores the importance of building orientation.[108]

In relation to *valetudinaria*, the only structural comment made by Hyginus about such buildings was that they should be positioned where '*there may be quiet*'.[109] And there is certainly evidence that, among hospital patients today, noise is associated with high blood pressure and worse rates of recovery from heart attacks. Ulrich argues that a quiet hospital is created mainly through appropriate design of the physical environment, not by modifying staff behaviour or organisational culture.[110]

CHAPTER 5

Pharmaceutical Remedies

Pharmaceutical remedies had a long pedigree prior to the advent of the Greek or the Roman civilisations. The oldest documentary evidence for the use of medicinal plants for the preparation of drugs has been found on a Sumerian clay tablet dated to around 3000 BC. Subsequently, the Egyptian Ebers Papyrus – from 1550 BC – provided details of numerous herbal treatments.[1]

Homer's epics from the eighth century BC – the Iliad and the Odyssey – mention sixty-three plant species from Minoan, Mycenaean, Egyptian and Assyrian pharmacology. Four hundred years later, the works of Hippocrates contain three hundred medicinal plants and Theophrastus in *De historia plantarum* around five hundred. Examples of commonly used ancient remedies included garlic, mandrake, wormwood, fig and pomegranate. The male fern root seems to have been a particularly effective treatment against tapeworms – probably due to the presence of the chemical filicin.[2]

Today, we think of a drug as any substance that causes a change in a person's physiology or psychology in contrast to a food that provides nutritional support. But many items derived from plants or animals could serve as both foods and medicines. It might be that our ancestors observed that some foods had specific effects on the body and then applied these properties medically. Galen sought to differentiate foods from drugs by considering the mode of action, writing: '*now those substances which are assimilated are called foods, all others are called drugs*'.[3] But the distinction between a medicine and a food is often not clear cut and this needs to be borne in mind in any consideration of ancient remedies. For example, garlic was viewed as a powerful treatment for a wide range of conditions as well as an important element in cooking.[4]

The Roman pharmacopoeia

The major surviving sources of information on the pharmaceutical remedies being used during the first and second centuries AD are contained in the writings of Scribonius Largus, Dioscorides, Celsus, Pliny the Elder and Galen. Supplementary evidence is provided by inscriptions on the small stones used to emboss eye medications (collyrium stamps) in addition to occasional archaeological finds of actual drugs.

Little is known of the life of Scribonius Largus, but it seems likely that he penned his major pharmaceutical work, *Compositiones medicamentorum* (*The Composition of Remedies*), during the period 43–48 AD. At the time, he was probably in Britain as part of Claudius' retinue and wrote:

> *You will, however, forgive me if at present I describe only a few compounds to you and have not written of all diseases, for as you know we are abroad and therefore only have a moderate number of books.[5]*

But, despite this inconvenience, his collection ran to 271 chapters covering treatments within every part of the body from head to toe. He also wrote specific sections on anti-toxins, plasters and poultices, and his 300 remedies were based on 242 plants, 36 minerals and 27 animal products.[6] Scribonius Largus provided the first clear account of opium and it is mentioned 33 times within *Compositiones medicamentorum*. In addition to commenting on its use as an analgesic, he described how it is made '*from the milk of the heads of wild poppies*'. He also outlined both the symptoms and the treatment of acute opium intoxication.[7]

Dioscorides was a first-century physician who served in the Roman army during the time of Nero. His military position and extensive travels provided opportunities for studying diseases in addition to collecting and identifying numerous pharmaceutical remedies. In his five books that constituted *De materia medica* (*On Medical Material*), he recorded many plants previously unknown to Greek and Roman physicians and tried to describe not only their qualities and remedial effects, but also something of their morphology – including roots, foliage and flowers. In all, he outlined 944 remedies of which 657 are plants or products derived from plants.[8]

Pliny the Elder, a contemporary of Dioscorides, wrote about approximately 1,000 medicinal plants in his books *Naturalis historia* (*Natural History*).[9] He even described a specific treatment for possible scurvy using

> *the plant known as the 'britannica,' which is good, not only for diseases of the sinews and mouth, but for quinsy also, and injuries inflicted by serpents. This plant has dark oblong leaves and a swarthy root. The Frisii, a nation then on terms of friendship with us, and within whose territories the Roman army was encamped, pointed out this plant to our soldiers: the name given to it, however, rather surprises me, though possibly it may have been so called because the shores of Britannia are in the vicinity, and only separated by the ocean.*[10]

Somewhat intriguingly, at Haltern in Northern Germany, a lid of a lead box was unearthed in 1928 inscribed with the words '*EX RADICE BRITANICA*' translated as '*extract of the root of Britannica*'.[11] It is tempting to imagine that the complete box would have held Pliny's remedy.

Pliny the Elder probably wrote much of his *Naturalis historia* during the reigns of Vespasian and Titus and, also, while he was governor of *Hispania Tarraconensis*. He was one of a group of writers who flourished in the early empire termed 'encyclopaedists'. Across several fields of human endeavour and achievement, they took it upon themselves to collect, consolidate and comprehensively record all the available knowledge in Latin.[12] Another first-century medical encyclopaedist, Celsus, was probably born about 25 BC and lived under the reign of Tiberius. In his *De medicina* (*On Medicine*), he discussed around 250 medicinal plants in addition to a wide range of inorganic medications based on, for example, copper, aluminium, arsenic, zinc, calcium, lead, iron, antimony and sulphur.[13] However, unlike Pliny, Celsus might have actually been a physician – he certainly demonstrates considerably greater technical understanding and a more critical approach to assessing information.[14]

Galen wrote extensively about the use of drugs, drawing widely from compilations by others such as the Cretan physician Andromachus the Elder and Asclepiades Pharmacion in addition to numerous lesser known figures across the Empire such as Axius (doctor in the British Fleet) for an eye medication. His major works were *The Properties of Simples*, *Antidotes* and two dealing with compound drugs. In all, he lists around 440 different plants and 250 other substances used as remedies with, in many cases, a wealth of information on issues such as storage, use and application.[15]

In addition to being an avid collector of recipes, Galen had access to a much broader range of ingredients by virtue of his residence in Rome together with his imperial associations. He used his range of contacts – including friends and officials – to procure substances from across the Empire. He also travelled widely himself and described visits to the mines of Soloi on Cyprus, the shores of the Dead Sea, and two trips to the island of Lemnos to obtain components for specific pharmaceutical recipes.[16]

The first medicines that had been developed by the ancients often consisted of a single ingredient, occasionally with an additive to counter any adverse effects such as a bitter taste or, perhaps, to improve appearance or preservation. But, during the early Roman period – and especially by the time of Galen – the emphasis was much more on using compound remedies made up of more than one active ingredient.

Andromachus the Elder, who was also physician to Nero, is credited with composing a formula for a drug made up of over 80 different components.[17]

The underlying humoral theory (see Chapter 2), applied by Galen to guide his pharmaceutical prescriptions, proposed that each substance being used for treatment had both basic and derivative qualities. The basic qualities were the same for anything: active qualities (hot and cold) or passive qualities (dry and moist). The derivative qualities concerned the observable effects of a substance (such as a medication) on the body: heating or cooling, drying or moistening, but also actions such as mollifying, burning, purging, rotting or suppurating. In addition, it was necessary to consider the strength of the substance and whether it attracted a specific type of humour, which it then expelled from the body (i.e. as in the case of purgatives or emetics). In applying this theoretical foundation to select an appropriate drug, the physician also had to ascertain the nature of a patient's imbalance and the intensity of any therapeutic intervention required.[18]

Plant remains that might have had a role in medical treatment have been identified within various Roman archaeological contexts across Europe. Examples include celery, poppy, henbane, rue, cabbage and dock. However, although all these were promoted as therapies by Greco-Roman medical authors, such bio-archaeological finds need to be treated with great caution.[19] Although cabbage (found at Vindolanda) was recommended as both a laxative and a poultice, there is simply no evidence that the remains identified served either of these purposes. The faecal matter in the sewers at Bearsden on the Antonine Wall contained seeds of celery (used to improve urine output) and opium poppy but, again, this indicates only that the substances were ingested, not why they were ingested.[20] Opium was used as a culinary flavouring as well as an analgesic.

Also, if we accept that medication and dietary modifications were equally important approaches to treatment by most Roman physicians, this adds another level of uncertainty to the organic finds. Thus, even if the imported figs found in London and Silchester were 'medical', they might have been for treating a patient by dietary modification rather than, as suggested by Celsus, cooked over charcoal and then specifically used for coughs and sore throats.[21]

In addition to being drunk for enjoyment, wine was an important vehicle for medication. According to Dioscorides, Celsus and Pliny, horehound was frequently used to treat chest complaints and a shard of an amphora inscribed *prasi[on]* (horehound) in Greek letters has been discovered at Carpow in Scotland. The Aminean wine that found its way to Caerleon within an amphora marked '*AMINE*' might have been used as a treatment for diarrhoea if taken with wheat and bread.[22]

Therapies based on arsenic are occasionally encountered within the Greco-Roman pharmacopoeia. Realgar, orange-red crystals of arsenic sulphide, was recommended by Celsus as an antiseptic for the cleansing of wounds and ulcerations. In 1895, several lumps of realgar were discovered within the Roman town of Silchester but whether this find represents a medicine or a paint remains an open question.[23]

Associated archaeological artefacts can sometimes assist by providing a more 'medical' context for discoveries. For example, found alongside the remains of herbs from the Roman military hospital in Neuss in Germany were various implements that might have been used for grinding them into powder for use in prescriptions (see Chapter 4). The examination of residues from cylindrical bronze medical instrument containers held in the British Museum has identified beeswax, fat, conifer resin and gum-derived sugars, plus lead and zinc salts.[24]

Eye remedies

Nowadays, eye complaints constitute about 2 per cent of all patient encounters in UK general practice with conjunctivitis and corneal abrasions accounting for over half. However, in the ancient world it seems likely that eye problems were considerably more prevalent, possibly exacerbated by poorer hygiene practices (see Chapter 3). Crowded bathhouses and the excellent communications afforded by the road network would undoubtedly have contributed to the spread of infectious eye diseases (see Chapter 4).

Within the Roman medical literature there is a significant emphasis on the treatment of a variety of eye diseases using eye ointments – or collyria. For example, Scribonius Largus mentioned 22 collyria and Galen over 200. In *De medicina*, Celsus devoted a whole chapter to ophthalmology. Further information derives from the small stone stamps used to mark an individual collyrium with the name of the maker and the purpose of an eye treatment (see Chapter 3). The inscriptions on the stamps generally comprise two or three of the following elements: the medicament(s); a personal name (usually in the genitive case); and the nature of the ailment(s) or indication(s) for use.[25]

Lippitudo (conjunctivitis) is the mostly frequently cited problem being mentioned on eleven of the British stamps. The example from Cambridge is inscribed on one face:[26]

L. IVL. SALVTARIS PE/NICILLUM AD LIPPITUD

the collyrium of Lucius Julius Salutaris, to be applied with a fine brush for lippitudo of the eyes

On a second side is:

MARINI CAES

the collyrium named caesarianum according to the recipe of Marinus.

Caesarianum was known to Celsus who indicated that it could certainly be used for *lippitudo* and consisted of shoemaker's blacking (probably copper/iron sulphide), misy (probably iron/copper pyrites), white pepper, opium, gum, cadmia (zinc carbonate) and stibium (antimony sulphide). The St Albans stamp prescribes 'a *salve of myrrh to be used twice a day with egg'* for *lippitudo* and the Cirencester stamp is inscribed *'Minervalis's salve of frankincense for the onset of lippitudo, to be used with an egg'*.[27]

Examination of all the eye stamp inscriptions found across the Western Empire by Jacques Voinot reveals a variety of organic and inorganic components including vinegar, opium poppy, saffron, frankincense, myrrh, ox gall, nard and aloe, in addition to several metallic compounds based on iron (e.g. haematite), aluminium (e.g. alum), lead (e.g. cerussa and psimithium), mercury (e.g. cinnabar), zinc (cadmia and spodii) and copper (e.g. aerugo, stomoma, aes ustum, flos aeris and lepidum). Cadmia (zinc carbonate) and the latex of the opium poppy (lachryma papaveris) were particularly common constituents.[28]

In 1854 a possible Roman doctor's grave from Rheims was discovered and found to contain nineteen medical instruments together with the reasonably well-preserved remains of several collyria. Chemical analyses at the time of some of these revealed that they consisted of organic components combined with significant amounts of metallic compounds: iron oxide (16%), copper oxide (4%), lead oxide (23%) and calcium carbonate (17%).[29]

More recently – in 1990 – another probable doctor's tomb dated to the first century AD was excavated just outside Lyon. The cremated remains of the occupant were associated with a rectangular brass medicine box containing twenty sticks of dried collyria, a tubular case with three probes (of the type commonly used to mix and apply medicaments) and a worn stone mixing palette.[30]

One clearly stamped collyrium bore the medication name *stratioticum* in Greek alongside the personal name of *Zmaragdos*; possibly the identity of the doctor in the grave. *Stratioticum* was described by Scribonius Largus as containing a variety of ingredients including cadmia, pepper, psimithium, opobalsamum and opium.[31] It was therefore fascinating to discover that, on chemical analysis, this particular collyrium was rich in zinc carbonate (cadmia) and lead carbonate (psimithium) in addition to various organic elements.

Over three hundred years after the death of Scribonius Largus, the Gallo-Roman physician Marcus Empiricus also mentioned *stratioticum*, indicating that this remedy had survived the passage of time, albeit with some minor modifications. As in the case of the *Zmaragdos* collyrium, Marcus Empiricus' formulation included a small amount of chalcitidis (a combination of iron and copper salts) and he recommended it as 'a *good remedy for swellings in the eyes and for stopping stinging tears, for rough eye-lids and for blurred vision and scars which stem from the dust and smoke of the roads*'.[32]

Another collyrium from Lyon inscribed *dialibanum* was found to contain salts of copper, zinc, arsenic, antimony, iron and lead in addition to gum Arabic, myrrh and significant amounts of Euphrasia officinalis pollen. Celsus described *dialibanum* as consisting of '*roasted and washed copper, and parched poppy-tears 4g each; washed zinc oxide, frankincense, roasted and washed, antimony sulphide, myrrh, and gum 8g each*'.[33] The slight discordance between the recipes of Celsus and Zmaragdos might, perhaps, as in the case of *stratioticum*, reflect the modification of some compound medicines over time or by geographical location.

Other finds of Greco-Roman medicines come from the contents of a probable medical chest found among the cargo of a shipwreck off Pozzino in Italy. The excavators uncovered a cache of tin pyxides (cylindrical boxes often used to hold medicines or cosmetics) and box wood vials (5–6cm × 2cm) alongside a small stone moratorium, an iron probe and a bronze cupping vessel [Plate 25]. Within one of the tin pyxides, five grey discoid tablets were discovered with diameters of around 4cm. Although it is unclear whether these were eye collyria, it seems certain that they were ancient medicines based on their appearance and the context in which they were found. Analysis of the tablets revealed zinc as the main element (75%) along with silicon (9%) and iron (5%). The associated plant remains included starch grains in addition to significant amounts of pollen from *Olea europaea* (olive) and *Centaurea nigra* (knapweed). DNA sequencing has also revealed that the medicines contained carrot, radish, parsley, celery, wild onion and cabbage.[34]

What can the Romans teach us today?

For many generations after the fall of the Western Empire, Roman remedies continued to be used. In the late sixteenth century, the antiquary William Camden visited Hadrian's Wall and wrote:

> *The Roman souldiers of the marches did plant here every where in old time for their use, certain medicinable hearbes, for to cure wounds: whence it is that some Emperick practitioners of Chirurgery in Scotland, flock hither every yeere in the beginning of summer to gather such simples and wound herbes; the virtue whereof they highly commend as found by long experience, and to be of singular efficacy.[35]*

But, over the last couple of centuries, developments in chemistry and pharmacology combined with a paradigm shift in our thinking about how drugs might work have led to a loss of interest in ancient medicines.

For some doctors today, the Roman pharmacopoeia is now simply viewed as a source of amusing anecdotes about ridiculous or outlandish approaches to treatment. Scribonius Largus' comments on the use of the liver of a freshly killed gladiator to treat epilepsy are frequently cited.[36] In addition, mention is often made of the Roman penchant for bizarre recipes such as roasted seahorses or boiled mice to help incontinence, various animal dungs as therapies to cure warts and gout, or chameleon soaked in wine to treat headaches.[37]

At the other extreme, some of my medical colleagues seem to be under a mistaken impression that the Romans were instrumental in developing some of the basic treatments that we still use today. This perception is often founded on an over-optimistic interpretation of the ancient literature or relying on secondary sources of information. For example, it has been suggested that the ancients had a form of aspirin as they harnessed various parts of the willow (*salix alba*) for medical purposes. But, what Dioscorides actually wrote was that '*the juice from the leaves and bark warmed with rosaceum in a cup of malum punicum [pomegranate] helps sores in the ears, and a decoction of them is an excellent warm pack for gout*'.[38] And Celsus simply described the use of willow in the context of treating a prolapsed womb: '*After being treated in one of these ways, it is to be replaced, and pounded plantain or willow leaves boiled in vinegar applied*'.[39] Pliny also recommended a '*decoction of the bark and leaves in wine*' for gout but only suggested taking willow leaf extract by mouth to '*check over-lustful desire*'.[40]

However, there are things that the Romans can still teach us today in identifying new medicines in addition to helping us to use our existing therapies more wisely.

Identifying new medicines

On the face of it, it would seem odd that advanced civilisations such as the Egyptians, Greeks or Romans would use, and continue to use, the same medications over many hundreds of years if they were totally ineffective. Galen certainly selected remedies that had survived the passage of time and been assessed by experience – both of a particular physician and of a long tradition of doctors. Even today Roman remedies that some of my patients still use include cabbage and Euphrasia officinalis eye drops.

The Roman writer Cato suggested applying raw cabbage '*as a poultice on all kinds of wounds and swellings; it will cleanse all sores and heal without pain*',[41] and this is a treatment still occasionally recommended for women with breast discomfort associated with infant feeding. Moreover, modern research has demonstrated that cabbage leaves used for breast engorgement reduces pain and breast hardness in addition to increasing the duration of breast feeding.[42] One of the eye medicines unearthed from Lyon contained significant amounts of Euphrasia officinalis pollen.[43] Although this remedy is not mentioned by Galen, Pliny or even Dioscorides, Euphrasia has been

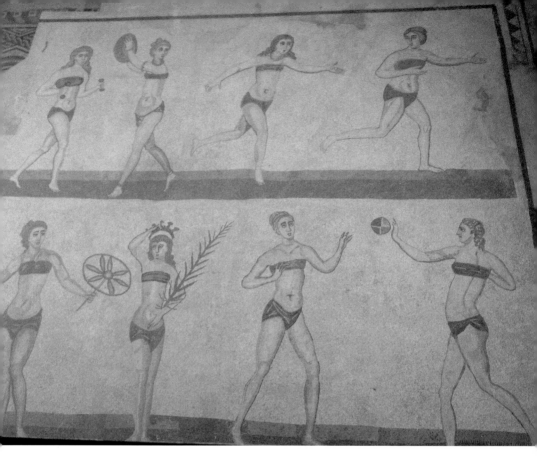

Plate 1. Gymnasium scene mosaic, Villa Romana del Casale, Sicily.

Plate 2. The boat-shaped prow, including staff and serpent relief, at the Aesculapian site on Tiber Island.

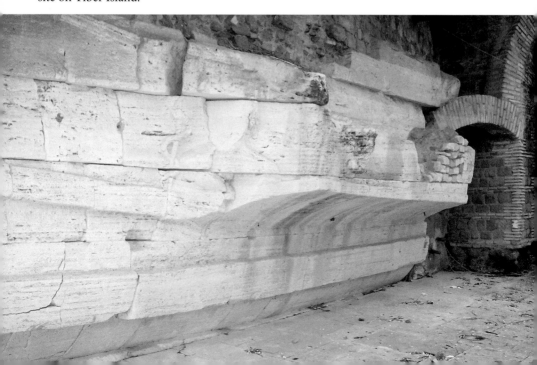

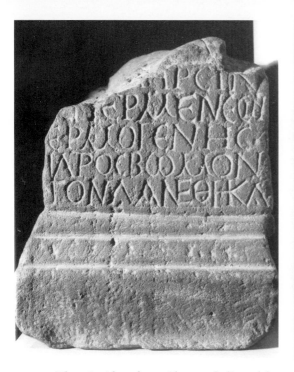

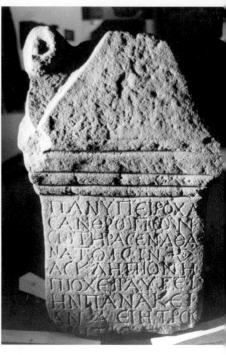

Plate 3. Altar from Chester dedicated by the Greek physician Hermogenes.

Plate 4. Altar from Chester dedicated by the Greek physician Antiochus.

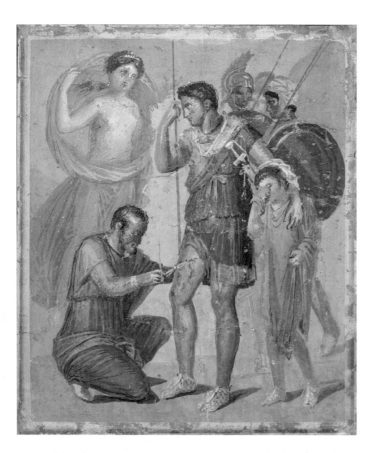

Plate 5. Wall-painting from Pompeii showing wounded Aeneas having an arrowhead removed.

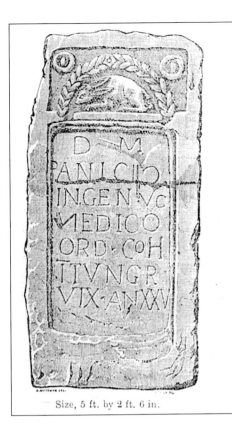

```
D  M
A N I C I O
I N G E N V O
M E D I C O
O R D . C O H
I T V N G R
V I X . A N X X V

Diis  Manibus
Anicio
Ingenuo
Medico
Ordinario (?)  Cohortis
Primæ  Tungrorum
Vixit  annos  viginti  quinque
```

Size, 5 ft. by 2 ft. 6 in.

Plate 6. Tombstone of Ancinus Ingenuus, *medicus ordinarius,* from Housesteads.

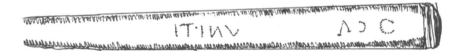

Plate 7. An inscribed bronze spatula from Caerleon belonging to Manilianus.

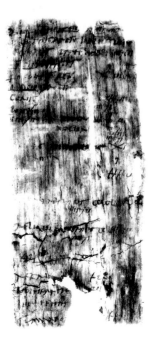

Plate 8. A writing tablet from Vindolanda reporting the strength of the First Cohort of Tungrians.

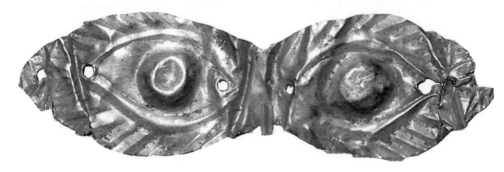

Plate 9. A pair of votive sheet-gold eyes unearthed at Wroxeter.

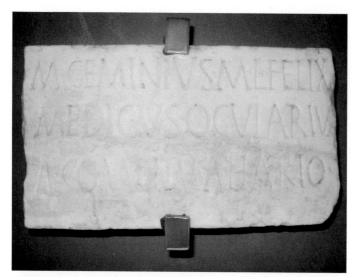

Plate 10. An inscription of a *medicus ocularis,* found in Rome.

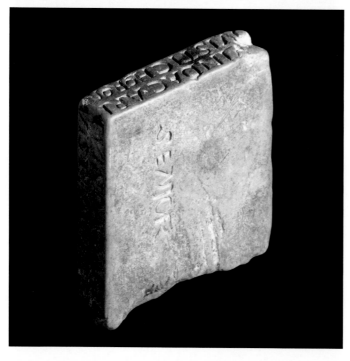

Plate 11. A collyrium stamp from Kenchester.

Plate 12. A collyrium stamp from Wroxeter.

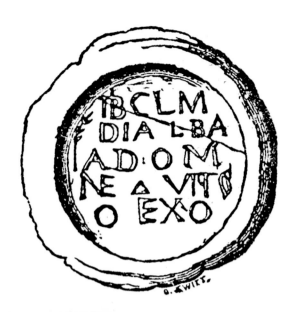

Plate 13. Marble tombstone of an Athenian physician, Jason.

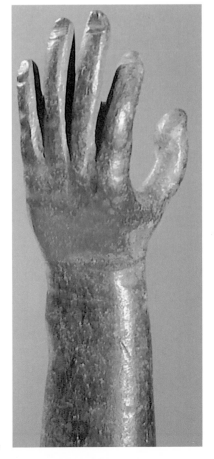

Plate 14. Votive forearm from Lydney.

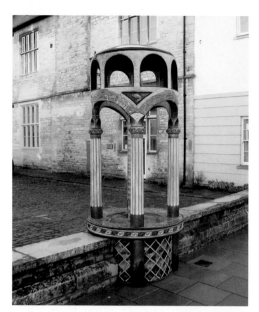

Plate 15. The modern fountain at the end of the Dorchester aqueduct.

Plate 16. The Lincoln aqueduct pipeline.

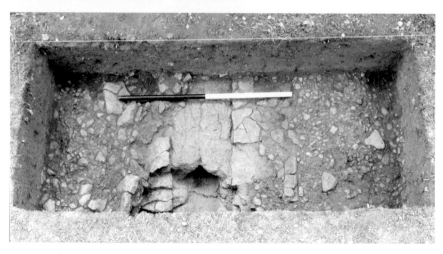

Plate 17. A view of the Dorchester aqueduct.

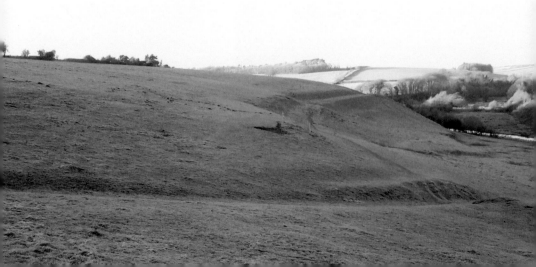

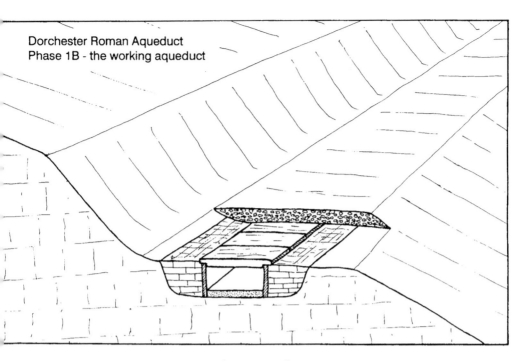

Dorchester Roman Aqueduct
Phase 1B - the working aqueduct

Plate 18. Cross-section of the Dorchester aqueduct.

Plate 19. Remains of the latrine at Housesteads.

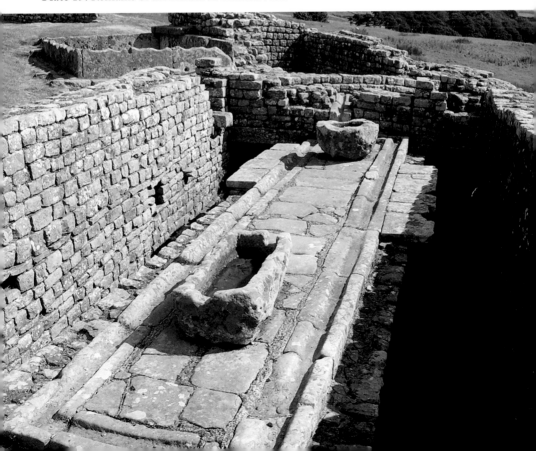

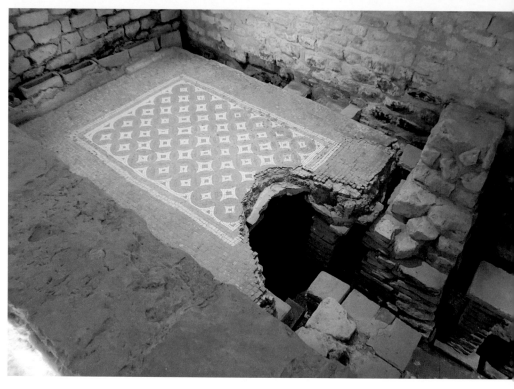

Plate 20. The *tepidarium* at Chedworth villa.

Plate 21. The hot spring water at Bath.

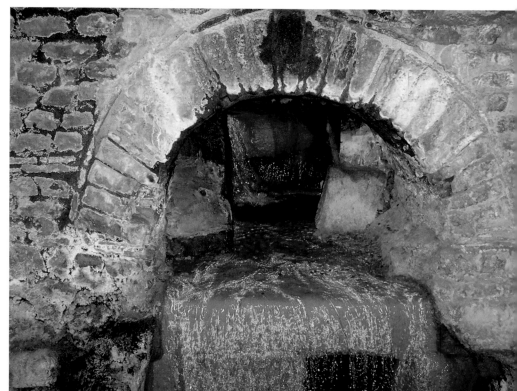

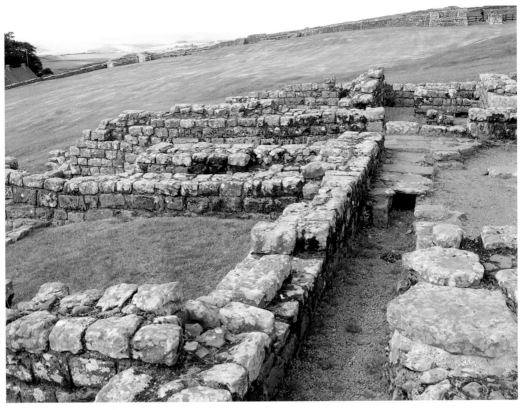

Plate 22. The hospital at Housesteads.

Plate 23. The drain leading from the latrine at Housesteads hospital.

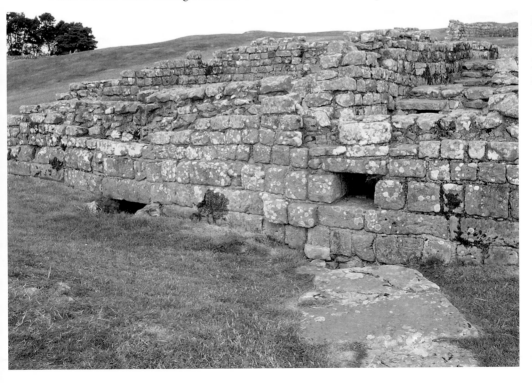

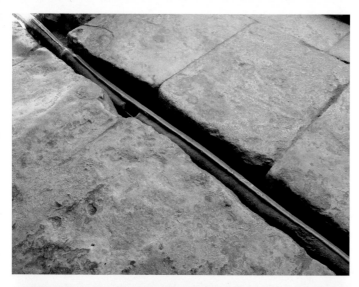

Plate 24. Roman lead piping at the Great Bath in Bath.

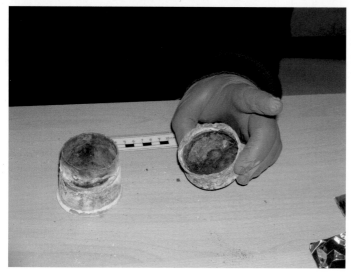

Plate 25. Tin pyxide from Pozzino containing ancient medication.

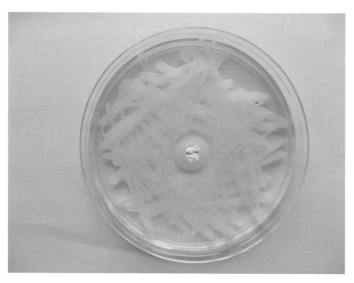

Plate 26. *Philo* collyrium in the centre of a Petri dish, with a circular bacteria 'kill zone' around the collyrium.

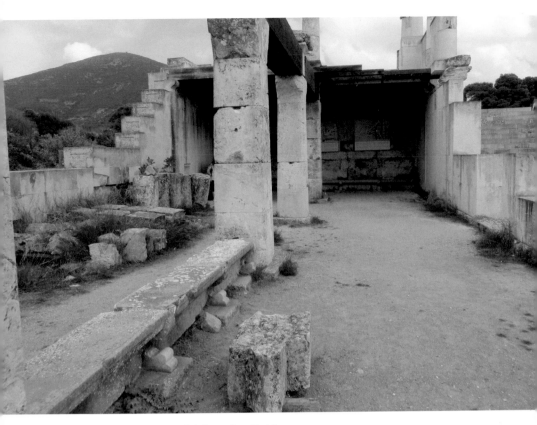

Plate 27. The 'dream room' (*abaton*) at Epidaurus.

Plate 28. Entrance to the Temple of Nodens at Lydney.

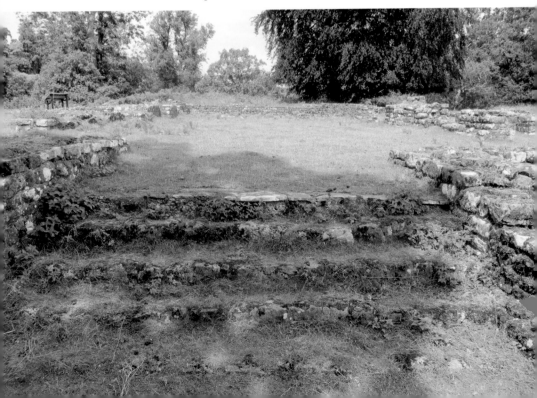

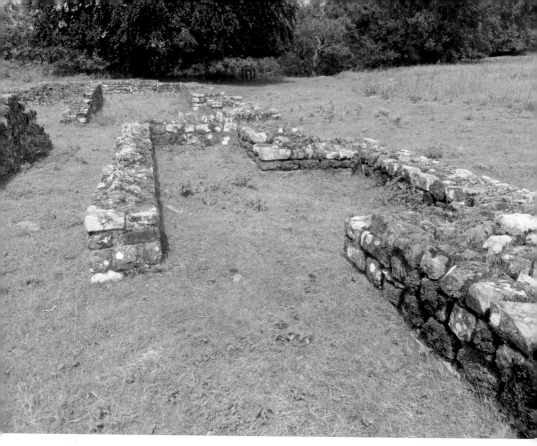

Plate 29. A probable 'dream room' (*abaton*) within the Temple of Nodens at Lydney.

Plate 30. The bathhouse at Lydney.

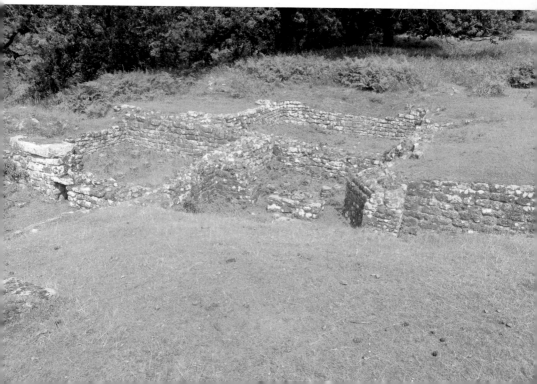

Plate 31. Bronze statuette of a dog, from Lydney (reproduction).

Plate 32. The theatre at Epidaurus.

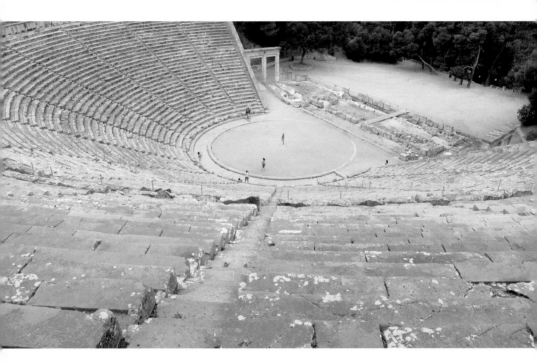

Plate 33. The prospect from the healing sanctuary at Corinth.

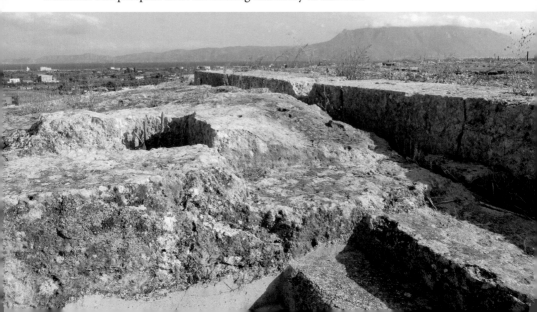

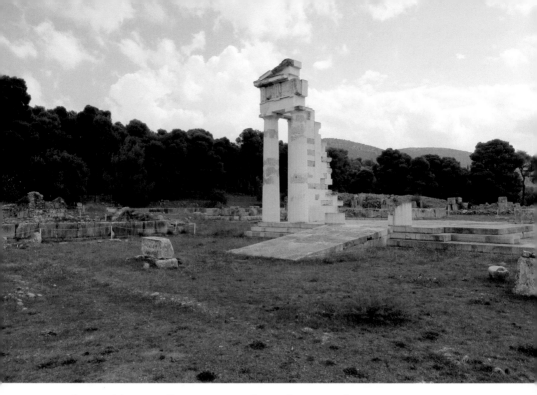

Plate 34. The partially-reconstructed *propylaea* at Epidaurus.

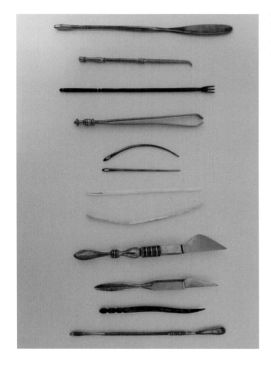

Plate 35. Reconstructed basic medical kit: forceps, needles (bone and brass), scalpels, probes and skin hooks.

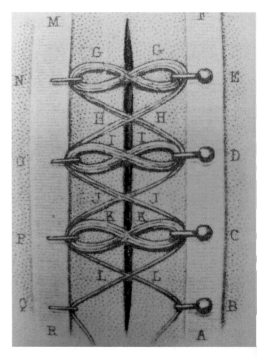

Plate 36. The use of *fibulae* for skin closure.

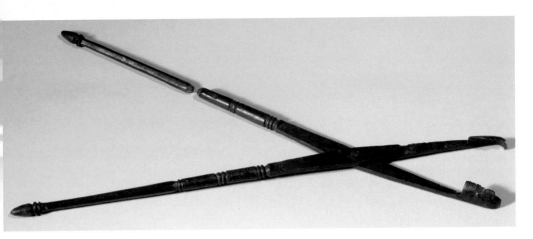

Plate 37. Uvula forceps (*staphylagra*) from Caerwent.

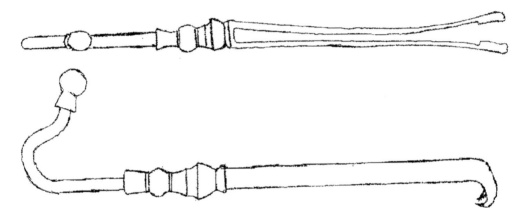

Plate 38. Brass surgical forceps from Littleborough.

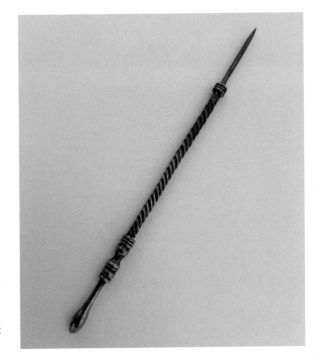

Plate 39. Reproduction cataract needle.

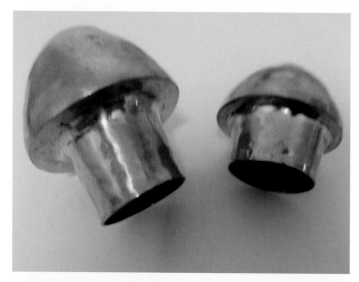

Plate 40. Reproduction cupping vessels.

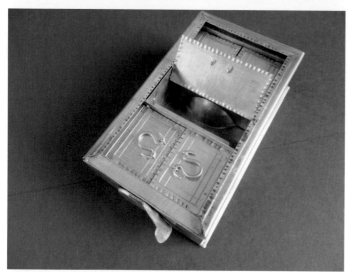

Plate 41. Reconstructed eye box with view of central compartment.

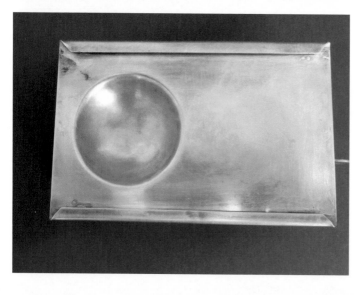

Plate 42. Cup-shaped depression on underside of reconstructed eye box.

used to treat sore, dry or red eyes for centuries and is still a major constituent of some homeopathic eye drops.

There is also evidence for the rediscovery of drugs mentioned in the ancient literature that have been long forgotten. For example, in relation to arthritic hip pain, Celsus wrote that: '*Inula root also pounded and afterwards boiled in dry wine and applied widely over the hip is among the most efficacious of remedies*'.[44] Boiling Inula helenium roots is known to release the chemical inulin and, in 2016, a patent was lodged focusing on the use of inulin sulphate for treating osteoarthritis.[45] It is unclear whether the applicants were aware of the earlier work by Celsus.

Since the mid-1990s, it has been possible to prescribe pain relief to patients in the form of self-adhesive skin patches incorporating strong analgesics such as Fentanyl or Buprenorphine. At the time, it was thought this was a major innovation in the management of pain, avoiding some of the side-effects associated with the oral treatments. But Galen's description of a formulation called '*Olympic Victor's Dark Ointment*' (OVDO) that could be applied extremally was intriguing as it combined opium with other elements – such as saffron – that might affect skin permeability. He stated that it was

useful for extreme pain, against eye swellings and an entirely appropriate eye collyrium since it provides relief immediately: cadmia (zinc carbonate) burnt & washed 8 drachma, acacia (gum Arabic) 8 drachma, stibii (antimony) burnt & washed 8 drachma, aloe Indica (aloe vera) 8 drachma, croci (saffron) 4 drachma, myrrh 4 drachma, opii (opium) 4 drachma, gummi (mastic) 8 drachma; mix with water and use with an egg. The mixture is thick. I also added 4 drachma of pompholygis (zinc oxide) and thuris (frankincense).[46]

It has been suggested that this treatment for pain and swellings might have been reserved for the winners of Olympic events who had sustained black eyes or other injuries during violent boxing or wrestling events. The key question was whether the ointment – when applied to the skin – could have acted as an effective analgesic by allowing opium to get into the body more easily? To answer this, Adrian Harrison and his colleagues diligently followed Galen's recipe for OVDO producing a viscous ointment that attached firmly to the skin as an elastic plaster-like layer. They then measured the amount of opium (morphine) that passed through abdominal mouse skin by raw opium solutions in comparison with the OVDO mixture. While hardly any morphine was able to penetrate the skin from the opium solutions, a considerable amount moved across when the opium was part of the OVDO formulation. Clearly, there is something about the combination that made OVDO a very effective transdermal analgesic.[47]

Infections and infectious diseases were common problems in the Roman world (see Chapter 4). Some of the descriptions of illnesses are so clear that, even today, it is quite possible to identify several conditions with considerable precision. For example, Galen's reports on individuals suffering from the Antonine Plague leaves many modern doctors in little doubt that they had smallpox.[48] Also, a lot of therapies were directed at treating infective conditions and one of these – honey – is playing an increasingly important role again today.

Honey is a complex mixture containing a variety of substances including fructose, glucose, proteins, amino acids, vitamins, minerals, antioxidants and organic acids. Dioscorides wrote that *'honey is cleansing, opens pores, and draws out fluids. As a result it is good for all rotten and hollow ulcers when infused. Boiled and applied it heals flesh that stands separated'*.[49] And, in relation to the care of wounds, Celsus stated that they *'must be cleaned. And this is best done by putting on lint soaked in honey'*.[50]

Recent research has revealed that honey can inhibit the growth of around 60 species of bacteria in addition to some fungi and viruses. It has also been successfully used to eradicate Methicillin-resistant Staphylococcus aureus (MRSA) from chronic wounds and to treat diabetic foot ulcers in addition to neutralising any foul odours.[51] The healing properties of honey were clearly demonstrated in a study comparing it against the standard treatments for burn victims. The results showed that honey treatments produced greater sterility of the wounds, a faster rate of healing, and a more rapid onset of healing. These experiments also indicated that wild honey was superior to artificial honey (which omits many of the 'non-sugar' components contained in wild honey).[52]

In analysing the available information on the commoner constituents of the Roman eye collyria, it is clear that many remedies contained antiseptics in one form or another. For example, the vinegar lotion of Gaius Valerius Amandus or the copper oxide within Aurelius Polychronius's collyrium might have been very effective anti-bacterials either in treating conjunctivitis or in preventing a corneal scar becoming infected while it healed. The collyrium of the British eye doctor Axius, referred to by Galen, probably also had many anti-microbial components in terms of its metallic constituents: copper oxide, zinc oxide, zinc carbonate and mercuric sulphide.[53]

Sally Pointer and I have manufactured and tested a modified version of the Philo collyrium described by Celsus. The ingredients used were equal parts (4g each) of cerussa (lead acetate), spodii (zinc oxide) and gum arabic. We carefully followed Celsus' instructions in '*pounding each of the ingredients separately and then mixed together gradually adding water*'.[54] It was fascinating to discover that the *Philo* collyrium exhibited the same microbiological efficacy (in vitro) as does one of the most commonly prescribed ophthalmological antibiotics – fusidic acid.[55] Plate 26 demonstrates the bacterial 'kill zone' around the *Philo* collyrium.

Much more advanced work on possible ancient anti-microbials has been undertaken by Freya Harrison and her colleagues at the University of Nottingham using Bald's Leechbook. This is a large collection of Anglo-Saxon medical recipes written in the tenth century with many of the remedies being derived from Roman authors including

Pliny, Galen, Celsus, Oribasius and Marcellus Empiricus. One of the particularly interesting features of Bald's Leechbook is the focus of several treatments on clearly recognisable infective conditions. For example, the recipe for wen (sty) is described as follows:

Make an eye salve against a wen: take equal amounts of cropleac (an allium species) and garlic, pound well together, take equal amounts of wine and oxgall, mix with the alliums, put this in a brass vessel, let (the mixture) stand for nine nights in the brass vessel, wring through a cloth and clarify well, put in a horn and at night apply to the eye with a feather; the best medicine.[56]

This formulation was carefully reconstructed and its ability to neutralise the bacterium Staphylococcus aureus was then examined. Not only did the resulting mixture destroy bacteria in a laboratory planktonic culture but it also worked on an in vitro model of a soft tissue infection (known as a synthetic biofilm). Moreover, the eye salve eliminated MRSA from mice with chronically infected wounds. A particularly fascinating finding was that, although it was recognised that many of the individual components of the remedy had anti-bacterial properties, the effect of the whole was greater than the sum of the parts. Therefore, the overall anti-microbial activity might be dependent on a cocktail of substances working in different ways to destroy bacteria, or there may be specific chemical processes occurring during the preparation that magnify the effects of the individual ingredients.[57]

Dioscorides, Pliny, Celsus, Galen and Scribonius Largus all mentioned the use of Lemnian earth from the island of Lemnos as a treatment. This is a complex material consisting of clay minerals (montmorillonite, kaolin) together with alum (20%) and haematite (5%). Galen wrote that:

whenever I have used Lemnian earth in malignant and putrid ulcers it has proved to be of great value; its use is here determined by the size of the ulcerating surface. If this be fetid, and very boggy and foul, it is checked by Lemnian seal dissolved in very sour vinegar and brought to the consistence of mud.[58]

He also described the process for the preparation of Lemnian earth, the medication, from Lemnian earth, the raw material, as follows:

The priestess collects this, to the accompaniment of some local ceremony, no animals being sacrificed, but wheat and barley being given back to the land in exchange. She then takes it to the city, mixes it with water so as to make moist mud, shakes this violently and then allows it to stand. Thereafter she removes first the superficial water, and next the fatty part of the earth below this, leaving only the stony and sandy part at the bottom, which is useless. She now dries the fatty mud until it reaches the consistency of soft wax; of this she takes small portions and imprints upon them the seal of Artemis; then again she dries these in the shade till they are absolutely free from moisture.[59]

Over recent years, a considerable amount of work has been undertaken by Effie Photos-Jones and her colleagues on Lemnian earth. It certainly seems to be an effective anti-microbial and it is suggested that the process of enrichment described by Galen was important in maximising its effectiveness. Perhaps the alum and haematite act as the antibacterial and astringent components with the clay serving as a poultice to reduce swelling.[60]

Most of the antibiotics prescribed today are single compounds, and modern doctors are encouraged to avoid using combinations such as *Co-amoxiclav* or *Co-fluampicil*. Therefore, it is interesting to discover that some effective anti-microbials used by our ancient forebears (i.e. honey, Philo's collyrium, Bald's sty treatment and Lemnian earth) were not single simple substances but, rather, cocktails of different components. Perhaps their continuing effectiveness over many generations reflects the greater challenges for bacteria in developing resistance against treatments that attack them in multiple ways.

Identifying remedies from ancient sources is an area of growing interest spurred on by, for example, Tu Youyou's dramatic re-discovery of artemisinin to treat malaria.[61] The Nottingham-based *Ancientbiotics* consortium is now using bioinformatics tools combined with complex statistical analyses to examine ancient literature.[62] Their overarching objective is to find groups of ingredients that are combined in the same remedy and/or used to treat infection more often than expected by chance.

However, in mining ancient Roman texts to unearth any new treatments, there are important questions that need to be considered:[63]

1. What was the nature of the individual ingredient(s)?

Although identifying some ingredient(s) is straightforward, for others it can prove to be very tricky. Silphium is an example of a medicinal plant that was recommended by Hippocrates and used widely. It was described as having a think root, a stalk like a ferula and celery type leaves but, today, the exact nature of this plant remains elusive.[64] Sometimes it might only be possible to select a broad class for a likely ingredient or, even, a range of potential options. In manufacturing Bald's eye salve, it was unclear whether the component *'cropleac'* was onion or leek so both formulations were made up and evaluated.[65]

2. How were the ingredient(s) selected?

Consideration always needs to be given to how the ingredient(s) would have been selected. Nowadays, our focus might be on effectiveness and safety, but other issues may have been more influential in the choices made by Roman physicians such as the ease of obtaining certain items and/or their quality. Certain substances might have been unavailable to some doctors or found within specific localities leading to modifications. For example, one collyrium unearthed at Lyon was stamped '*crocodes*' indicating that it should have contained saffron but, although it might have been saffron-coloured, the biochemical analysis found no trace of saffron.[66] Celsus even stated that *'there are many collyria devised by many inventors, and these can be blended even now in novel mixtures, for mild medicaments and moderate repressants may be readily and variously mingled'*.[67]

In addition, some components – especially organic ones – might have rapidly deteriorated with storage and there was often little control over the quality of certain ingredients procured from drug sellers. Also, if a treatment was being used for a condition that might wax and wane or where a strong placebo effect was likely, then greater importance might have been attached to the taste, smell or outward appearance of a remedy.

3. How were the ingredient(s) prepared, combined and, if necessary, preserved for future use?

Although some authors provided the proportions for multiple ingredients in addition to the method of mixing/grinding and other details of preparation, or preservation, this is not always the case.

4. What disease or disorder was being targeted by the remedy?

In the ancient literature the identification of pathological entities was often imprecise with considerable diagnostic uncertainty. This is further compounded by how the words of any specific author have been translated and transmitted over the centuries.

Perhaps one of the advantages in focusing on remedies that might have an 'anti-infective' purpose is that precision is not as important as would be the case in trying to identify treatments for more specific conditions such as asthma or bowel cancer. As was evident from the work on Bald's remedy, treating a sty pointed towards the medicine being a possible ancient antibiotic and, once the formulation had been reconstructed, other anti-microbial therapeutic uses could then be explored such as its action against MRSA.[68]

5. How likely is a causal link between the treatment and any beneficial effects?

For some conditions it can be uncertain whether any improvement is based on the direct effects of a medicine or due to other factors such as the natural history of the condition being treated, the placebo effect, lifestyle changes (see Chapter 2) or any concomitant treatments. For example, Pliny commented that '*all the lettuces are believed to bring sleep*',[69] Dioscorides remarked that '*in general* [lettuce] *is sleep-inducing*'[70] and Celsus wrote that '*for producing sleep the following are good: poppy, lettuce, and mostly the summer kinds in which the stalk is very milky*'.[71]

Galen also stated that:

> *we see almost daily that wild lettuce, bathing in drinkable sweet and warm water, and the drinking of a wine moderately mixed with water, induce sleep as do all other substances which moisten and cool, but those of the opposite nature cause only sleeplessness.*[72]

Lettuce stems certainly contain lactucarium, which has mild narcotic properties and, in mice, has been demonstrated to increase sleep duration.[73] But there is also a strong placebo effect associated with sleep-inducing medications and, as indicated by Galen's comment, there are numerous other factors that can affect our sleep too.

6. How was the treatment prescribed?

Even if there is reasonable clarity about the pharmaceutical ingredients and the condition being treated, difficulties are frequently encountered in determining the precise method of application of a formulation, in addition to the dose, the frequency of use and the length of the course. But it might be that such imprecision was deliberate, encouraging cautious prescribing and allowing for a substantial margin of error.

It would then take a very significant overdose for the Roman physicians to put their patients (and themselves!) at any danger.

Improving the use of medicines

The Romans adopted a broad approach to medical care with pharmaceuticals being only one element (see Chapter 2). As Celsus stated:

> *medicine was divided into three parts, so that there was one which healed by regimen, another by drugs and a third manually. The Greeks named the first dietetics, the second pharmaceutics and the third surgery.*[74]

Scribonius Largus emphasised the importance of balance in ensuring that drug treatments are used appropriately *'freeing patients from pain and danger'*, going on to say that:

> *we must condemn those who try to eliminate the use of drugs from medicine whereas we must support those who want to help the patient with all possible means ... Indeed the physician helps patients by following certain steps. First he tries to treat by allowing the appropriate food at the appropriate time; then if the patient does not respond to this treatment medicaments are given.*[75]

Today, physicians have access to a much wider range of medicines than was the case for their Roman medical ancestors; but being able to prescribe more doesn't necessarily equate to better care. Across England around 17 per cent of adults are now taking long-term antidepressants and a further 13 per cent regular opioid-based pain medications but there is much more to the management of depression or a person's chronic pain than simply writing a prescription.[76] On the other hand,

and as pointed out by Scribonius Largus, there is a requirement to guard against underuse too by ensuring that individuals with, for example, high blood pressure, diabetes or heart disease are offered the best available medications. But even in these circumstances a balanced approach is still required with an emphasis on the features of hygiene as outlined in Chapter 2.

Roman doctors were certainly more cautious in their use of medications than is the case today. Part of this reticence might have been around uncertainties about the precise nature of the ingredients that a physician was able to procure from a drug seller. In relation to opium, Scribonius Largus implored his readers to:

make sure to use that which comes from the pulp of the poppy flower, not from the leaves, which the pedlars of ointments make for a profit. The former is wrought with great labour in small quantities; the other is ground up without bother and found abundantly.[77]

Galen also went to extraordinary lengths to assure the quality of his ingredients including, for example, travelling to Lemnos to observe how the medicinal clay was collected, washed, separated, dried and formed into small stamped seals.[78]

Nowadays, we are much more trusting about the medications we recommend or prescribe. But is our trust sometimes misplaced? Collectively, pharmaceutical businesses lose billions of pounds to counterfeit medications every year with significant numbers of associated deaths still occurring in countries with poor quality control, scant regulatory inspections, and a high demand for medicines. There are also frequent warnings about the dangers of purchasing some medications on-line.[79]

All medicines – ancient or modern – can cause harm if doctors don't focus on the individuality of the patient. Before writing a prescription, the physician needs to consider any treatments a person is already taking in addition to their age, gender, ethnic origin, other medical conditions, lifestyle and dietary habits. Such a personalised approach was promoted by the likes of Scribonius Largus, Galen and Celsus. Scribonius Largus emphasised the importance of selecting medicines that have been *'tested by use and experience'*[80] and Galen stated that

> *it is worthwhile for the doctor to know those that are discovered by experience alone and those that are discovered by theory alone. And third, in addition to these, there are those that came to discovery from both (experience and theory) jointly.*[81]

In his writings on Lemnian earth, Galen outlined that he had reviewed the existing evidence by getting a book from one of the islanders in *'which all the uses of Lemnian Earth were set forth'* before going away to test the medicine himself.[82] Such a rigorous approach based on assembling evidence, considering how the medicine might work (in accordance with humoral theory) and using his (and others') clinical experience remains a good model today. There will always be a requirement to ensure that doctors are basing their treatment decisions on sound evidence, a good theoretical understanding combined with significant clinical experience.

Although humoral theories have been replaced with more modern ideas about how the body works there is a need to appreciate that, as Galen indicated, theory alone can still let us down. For example, back in the 1980s patients who suffered from heart attacks were given medicines to regulate the heartbeat so as to prevent any sudden deaths. From a theoretical physiological perspective, this approach made complete sense but, unfortunately, it was subsequently discovered that rather than lowering death rates the medicines had the opposite effect.[83]

Those who rely on research findings alone and dismiss experience will also short-change their patients. Nowadays, we increasingly focus on data from randomised controlled trials to determine if a particular intervention works in terms of, for example, keeping people alive, curing disease, ameliorating symptoms such as pain or reducing disability. But a randomised controlled trial tells us that, on average, a medicine is of benefit to a certain group of patients. Some individuals will do better, and some will do worse than others. Also, some groups of people – especially the elderly and infirm – are never enrolled into such studies.[84]

Theory and evidence are important but, as recognised by our Roman forbears, experience still matters. There will always be a need to gauge if a drug works in the real world where things are a lot messier and variable than they are in a research setting.[85] Also, as in the Roman world, healers and patients must work together in deciding where the balance lies between the benefits and the harms of a medicine, as well as considering alternative options.

CHAPTER 6

Psychological Wellbeing and Holistic Care

In the Roman world, the distinction between physical and mental wellbeing was much more blurred than is the case today. Looking after the psyche – or the soul – was viewed as integral to the care of the body and it was a key element of Galen's *Hygiene* alongside movement, pure air, sleep and diet (see Chapter 2).

Galen also developed a particular interest in 'whole person' care including the interaction of the body and the soul. In his book on prognosis, *De praecognitione,* he devoted two of his detailed case histories to the identification and management of stress-related conditions – one a woman suffering from 'love sickness' and the other a slave with money worries. He then asked:

what was it that escaped the notice of earlier doctors who examined the aforesaid woman and slave? For such discoveries are made from common inductions, even if one has only the slightest acquaintance with medical science. I think that is because they have no clear conception of how the body tends to be affected by mental conditions, possibly they do not know also that the pulse is altered by strivings and fears that suddenly upset the mind.[1]

Many Romans citizens – in addition to physicians such as Galen – were seeking a philosophy of life. Their desire was to achieve tranquillity by addressing both the prevention and the treatment of a range psychological disturbances. One approach popularised by the likes of Seneca, Epictetus and Marcus Aurelius that found favour in the early Roman Empire was Stoicism. The overriding aim was to replace negative emotions such as grief, anger and anxiety with positive emotions such as joy.[2]

Other individuals, such as the Emperor Caracalla, frequented healing sanctuaries. These places focused on holistic care (including psychological wellbeing) by offering a broad range of treatments in addition to enlisting the assistance of healing deities, most notably Aesculapius.[3]

In the first of his six books on *Hygiene*, Galen wrote that:

> *not a few men, however many years they were ill through the disposition of their souls, we have made healthy by correcting the disproportion of their emotions. No slight witness of the statement is also our ancestral god Aesculapius who ordered not a few to have odes written as well as to compose comical mimes and certain songs.*[4]

On the face of it, it might seem odd that such a rational individual as Galen was also interested in divine cures. But, within the Roman world the focus was not simply about 'being cured' or 'surviving' but the broader concepts of 'healing' and 'growth'. These two sides of the therapeutic relationship might even be termed 'Hippocratic' and 'Aesculapian'.[5]

Many Greeks and the Romans were interested in dreams and, unlike us, they wrote about *seeing* a dream rather than *having* a dream. Divine beings appearing in such dreams were viewed as distinct entities, thereby allowing them to communicate with the dreamer in giving advice or guidance.[6] For example, Galen's entry into the medical profession was said to have been precipitated by a dream experienced by his father, Nicon. Subsequently, when Galen was twenty and afflicted by a subdiaphragmatic abscess, he reported that Aesculapius appeared to him in a dream with instructions to open an artery in his hand, thereby saving his life. Several years later, in another dream, Aesculapius forbade him to travel to war with the Emperor Marcus Aurelius.[7]

The second century orator Aelius Aristides was troubled by a series of illnesses throughout his life for which he sought relief at the shrines of Aesculapius. He left detailed records of such therapeutic experiences – including dream-healing – in his *Hieroi Logoi* (Sacred Tales).[8]

Stoicism

Galen was no stranger to loss. He was very close to his father, Nicon, who died when Galen was nineteen. The Antonine Plague then took away several friends in addition to all his slaves and, subsequently, a great fire consumed a large portion of his library (including many of his own works), medicines and possessions.[9] In his book *De tranquillitate animi* (*Avoiding Distress*), Galen reflected on these events and went on to write about how he coped with living under the brutal Emperor Commodus:

> *You yourself, I believe, are convinced that the crimes committed by Commodus in a few years are worse than any in the whole of recorded history. So when I saw all of these things happening daily, I schooled my imagination to prepare for the loss of everything that I had ... I also expected to be sent to a desert island, like other innocent victims ... I advise you to train your soul's imagination to cope with almost any turn of events.*[10]

Like many Romans of this time, Galen was particularly attracted to the Stoicism, based on the teachings of the Hellenistic philosopher Zeno (333–261 BC), writing:

> *We should be amazed, if at all, at those who are not upset even when they have lost everything, like Zeno of Citium, who, they say, at the report of a shipwreck in which he had lost everything, remarked, 'You've done us a favour, Fate, by driving us to the philosopher's cloak and the Stoa.'*[11]

Zeno's ideas were both taken up and modified by the Romans with a particular emphasis on the attainment of virtue and tranquillity. Virtue was about 'living in accordance with nature' and leading a 'good life' and this was seen as much more than simply making a good living (see Chapter 2). The emphasis was on existing as humans are designed to live – especially using the ability to reason and acting for the common good. The Stoics suggested that, although we share many instincts with other animals, our ability to think rationally is what makes us human.[12]

Some key individuals involved in the Romanisation of Zeno's Stoic philosophy were Seneca, Epictetus and Marcus Aurelius. They argued that a life plagued with negative emotions such as anger, anxiety (including social anxiety), grief, fear (e.g. of old age and dying) and envy would not be a good life. But the Roman Stoics also did not, unlike their fellow Cynics, spurn creature comforts.[13]

At the start of his handbook, the *Encheiridion*, Epictetus, a former slave, wrote:

> *Some things in the world are up to us, while others are not. Up to us are our faculties of judgement, motivation, desire, and aversion – in short, everything that is our own doing. Not up to us are our body and property, our reputations, and our official positions – in short, everything that is not our own doing. Moreover, the things that are up to us are naturally free, unimpeded, and unconstrained, while the things not up to us are powerless, servile, impeded, and not our own. Keep this is mind then: if you think things naturally servile are free and that things not our own are ours, you will be frustrated, pained and troubled, and you will find fault with gods and men.*[14]

Epictetus was making the point that most people thought that harms and benefits came from external factors and this is where they directed their attention. But, aiming to change the world around us to attain contentment was viewed by Epictetus as a sure route to dissatisfaction and unhappiness, as we are then striving for things that are not within our control. To attain tranquillity, the Stoics argued that it is better and easier for individuals to change themselves. Thus, although we might not have control over events, we can always control our reactions to such events. This involves working to suppress the desire to add a personal twist or to make inappropriate value judgements. As Epictetus explained: '*It is not things themselves that trouble people, but their opinions about things.*'[15] And Marcus Aurelius added that as we have it within our power to assign value to things, we also have it in our power to live a good life. He wrote: '*Everything is but what your opinion makes it; and that opinion lies with yourself. Renounce it when you will, and at once you have rounded the foreland and all is calm; a tranquil sea, a tideless haven.*'[16]

A particular challenge highlighted by Marcus Aurelius was desiring or seeking things that are not within our control such as fame, riches, immortality or reputation. There is a requirement to appreciate that life is unpredictable and most things that happen are not up to us, and he emphasised: '*Impermanence is the badge of each and every one; and yet you chase after them, or flee from them, as though they were to endure for all eternity.*'[17] Specifically in relation to other people's opinions and attitudes, he wrote: '*Begin each day by telling yourself: Today I shall be meeting with interference, ingratitude, insolence, disloyalty, ill-will, and selfishness – all of them due to the offenders' ignorance of what is good or evil.*'[18]

Healing sanctuaries

Religion was closely intertwined with all aspects of Roman life and, in appreciation of the limitations of terrestrial medicine, many individuals turned to the gods for help and guidance. Apollo was the original classical deity associated with medicine but, as time passed, Aesculapius (or Asclepius to the Greeks), the son of Apollo by Coronis, gradually became the divine being more clearly linked with health care. Aesculapius was born by Caesarean section and trained in medicine by the centaur Chiron. The young Aesculapius is also said to have been guarded by serpents and dogs – two animals that subsequently became associated with the Aesculapian creed. The offspring of Aesculapius included Acesis (Telesphorus), Hygieia (Salus) and Panacea.[19]

The original Aesculapian sanctuaries were established at Epidaurus, Cos and Pergamum with the first Roman temple to Aesculapius being built on Tiber Island [Plate 2]. Subsequently, the cult spread widely across the Empire being popularised by physicians in addition to the Roman army. Some sites were even patronised by emperors and, as a result, saw their standing increase leading to enrichment, revival and rebuilding. Hadrian certainly visited Epidaurus and Pergamon while, according to Dio Cassius, Caracalla tried out several.[20]

However, although Aesculapius and his family were associated with health, it would be wrong to assume that healing was dissociated from the other ancient gods. Healing prayers or health-seeking offerings could be directed at any deity according to the individual's preference. There was also evidence for religious syncretism with the blending of Roman beliefs and approaches with local gods. For example, Eshmun at Sidon (Lebanon), Nodens at Lydney and Sulis Minerva at Bath (UK), Apollo Grannus at Grand (France), Lennus Mars at Trier (Germany), Serapis and Isis at Canopus (Egypt) and the merging of Aesculapius with the Thracian horseman at Glava Panega (Bulgaria).[21]

The key facilities available at the major healing sites were a source of water – with wells, fountains and baths; temples; an *abaton* (dream room or dormitory), an area to exhibit votives and testimonials plus a space for exercising, rituals, festivals, and processions. Some also had libraries, theatres, banqueting halls, stadia, gymnasia and accommodation for visitors.[22] Sleeping in an *abaton* (or, in some situations, elsewhere in the sanctuary) and undergoing a process of ritual incubation was a central element of the Aesculapian healing process. During incubation, Aesculapius was said to appear in a dream-vision and either heal the individual directly or provide them with guidance about what was required to effect a cure.[23] However, sometimes the instructions were so cryptic that they required clarification by a member of the temple staff, the interpreter of dreams. For example, Aelius Aristides mentioned that *'when morning dawned, I call the physician Theodotus; and as he comes, I describe to him my dreams'*.[24] The process also involved priests and priestesses circulating among the sleepers with serpents and dogs, the curative dreams apparently being augmented by the touches of the clerics or the licks of the animals. Numismatic evidence suggests that the Aesculapian serpent was the species *Zamenis longissimus* and that the sacred dog resembled a hunting dog similar to an Irish wolfhound. In some cases, individuals might have been given specific narcotic drugs such as opium too.[25]

Although there was great variety in the size and location of *abatons* in the different Aesculapian sanctuaries, there were some features that held true for all of them. They had to be close to the temple with an easily accessible source of water, since incubants cleansed themselves upon entering the *abaton* and, at Pergamon, changed into white garments. Also, and perhaps most importantly, they had to be secluded and, at Epidaurus, it was a separate building near the temple, secured from one side by a wall and by a row of columns on the other [Plate 27]. In Roman times it had a two-storey extension to its western part, the lower level being enclosed by a wall and doors, and the upper by a stone balustrade.[26]

Undergoing incubation was not exclusive to the healing cult of Aesculapius. For example, Strabo described the use of healing dreams (both directly and indirectly) at a site dedicated to Pluto in Greece:

those who are diseased and give heed to the cures prescribed by the god resort thither and live in the village near the cave among experienced priests, who on their behalf sleep in the cave and through dreams prescribe the cures. These are also the men who invoke the healing power of the gods. And they often bring the sick into the cave and leave them there, to remain in quiet, like animals in their lurking-holes, without food for many days.

And sometimes the sick give heed also to their own dreams, but
still they use those other men, as priests, to initiate them into the
mysteries and to counsel them.[27]

At the sanctuary of Apollo Grannus at Grand (France) a dedicatory
inscription gives thanks for a cure *SOMNO IVSSVS* ... translated as '*after*
having received the order during his sleep'.[28] The Egyptian gods Serapis
and Isis also healed through dreams and the temple of Serapis on the
Greek island of Delos even employed professional dream interpreters.[29]

A detailed description of a contemporary visit to the Aesculapian
healing complex at Epidaurus in the second century AD was provided
by Pausanius:

The sacred grove of Aesculapius is surrounded on all sides
by boundary marks. No death or birth takes place within the
enclosure ... [Within the temple the statue of Aesculapius] is
sitting on a seat grasping a staff; the other hand he is holding
above the head of the serpent; there is also a figure of a dog
lying by his side ... Over against the temple is the place where
the suppliants of the god sleep. Near has been built a circular
building of white marble, called Tholos (Round House) ... In
it is a picture by Pausias representing Love ... and another
work, Drunkenness drinking out of a crystal cup ... Within the
enclosure stood slabs; in my time six remained, but of old there
were more. On them are inscribed the names of both the men and
the women who have been healed by Aesculapius, the disease
also from which each suffered, and the means of cure ... The
Epidaurians have a theatre within the sanctuary, in my opinion
very well worth seeing ... what architect could seriously rival
Polycleitus [the builder] in symmetry and beauty?.[30]

Based on various excavations undertaken during the last century,
the religious healing complex dedicated to Nodens at Lydney in

106

Gloucestershire was found to be extensive with many features similar the Aesculapian sanctuaries.[31] The temple itself was constructed with a central raised *cella* surrounded by an ambulatory or processional corridor. Projecting off this were several bays or chapels that may still be clearly seen today, as can the steps leading into the main entrance of the temple in the south-east [Plates 28 and 29]. Also, in the nineteenth century a mosaic was uncovered within the *cella* decorated with fish and sea monsters bearing the inscription: *D M N T FLAVIUS SENILIS PR REL EX STIPIBUS POSSUIT O[PITU] LANTE VICTORINO INTERP[RE]TIANTE* ... translated as '*for the god Mars Nodens, Titus Flavius Senilis, superintendent of the cult, from the offerings had this laid; Victorinus, the interpreter (of dreams), gave his assistance*'.[32]

Near to the temple stood three contemporary buildings: a square courtyard guest house to accommodate visiting worshippers, a well-equipped suite of baths, and a long narrow building containing many cubicles (*abaton*). Further to the north, a large water tank supplied the baths and the guest house [Plate 30].

Many items traditionally associated with healing cults have been found at Lydney. In addition to over 8,000 coins, 320 pins and 300 bracelets and brooches have been unearthed, perhaps gifts from women relieved of labour problems. There were also four inscriptions to the deity: two to Nodens equated with Mars, and two to Nodens alone. Unlike the Aesculapian temples in Greece, no representations of serpents (*Zamenis longissimus*) were found at Lydney, but rather nine statuettes of dogs in stone or bronze [Plate 31]. Perhaps such 'healing' dogs were more appropriate to Britain than the non-native 'healing' *Zamenis longissimus*. Certainly, from two testimonials found at Epidaurus, it is clear that both snakes and dogs could bring about cures by licking affected areas:

A man had his toe healed by a serpent. He, suffering dreadfully from a malignant sore in his toe, during the daytime was taken

107

outside by the servants of the temple and set upon a seat. When
sleep came upon him, then a snake issued from the abaton and
healed the toe with its tongue, and thereafter went back again
to the abaton.[33]

A dog cured a boy from Aegina. He had a growth on the neck.
When he had come to the god, one of the sacred dogs healed
him – while he was awake – with its tongue and made him well.[34]

There is evidence that a variety of more traditional and holistic treatments were provided at many healing sites alongside communing with the appropriate deity or undertaking dream healing/incubation. It was even suggested that Aesculapius could heal a patient directly (e.g. by laying on of hands, applying medicines or undertaking surgery) or indirectly by sending a dream in which he recommended a specific therapeutic regimen. Medical instruments have certainly been found at Epidaurus, Corinth and Lydney and there is evidence for the prescription of medications at Epidaurus.[35] Stamps for eye medicines have also been discovered at the sanctuaries of Nodens at Lydney and Sulis Minerva at Bath.[36]

Water was an extremely important element of many healing sites and was drunk for its healing properties as well as being used for bathing, hydrotherapy and ritual cleansing. Some sanctuaries, such as Bath (*Aquae Sulis*), were associated with hot springs or waters with specific mineral constituents[37] (see also Chapters 4 and 7). At Lydney, the iron rich nature of the waters might have encouraged individuals suffering from anaemia to visit based on the finding of a votive hand exhibiting koilonychia, a sign of iron-deficiency [Plate 14].[38] Aelius Aristides outlined the dramatic effects of using water from a well at the temple of Aesculapius at Pergamon:

For when bathed with it many recovered their eyesight, while
many were cured of ailments of the chest and regained their

necessary breath by drinking from it. In some cases it cured the feet, in others something else. One man upon drinking from it straightway recovered his voice after having been mute.[39]

Aside from having an emphasis on the principles of hygiene (see Chapter 2), a variety of arts-type therapies were probably practised at many of the ancient healing sites involving music, visual arts, reading and writing (including producing and reciting poetry) in addition to drama.[40] Arriving at Athens, Pausanius was particularly struck by the art works on display there, writing: '*The sanctuary of Aesculapius is worth seeing both for its paintings and for the statues of the god and his children. In it there is a spring.*'[41] The sights of soaring marbled buildings, sculptures, paintings and images of healing gods at many sites must have been quite a dramatic – and uplifting – experience for many visitors.

Hearing music and singing would also have been common experiences. Flute-playing is mentioned in a play by Athenaios and the remains of musical instruments have been found at several locations – including Lydney.[42] From Epidaurus and Pergamon there are reports of songs, hymns and even musical contests.[43] The physician Asclepiades of Bithynia treated various mental disorders by music, soporifics (wine) and exercise, specifically recommending that singing should be employed in the treatment of mania. Caelius Aurelianus wrote about the value of different varieties of piped music for symptoms of both anxiety and depression.[44]

Many healing sites boasted splendid theatres and the example at Epidaurus still enjoys perfect acoustics allowing an audience of up to 14,000 to hear actors without electronic amplification [Plate 32]. Such theatres would probably have been used for plays, celebrations of cures (including the singing of paeans), processions, festivals, games and choral performances. Viewing tragedies and comedies might also have formed part on an individual's treatment plan by putting their problems and worries into some sort of perspective.[45]

At some sites, the range of therapies could be broad – covering any condition and encompassing treatment in addition to prevention. In other places there might have been a specific focus on, perhaps, one area of the body or a specific problem. Based on an analysis of the anatomical votives found at the major sanctuaries, it seems likely that Athens specialised in ocular diseases while Corinth was the place for patients with limb injuries and genito-urinary problems. In Italy, the cult centre at Ponte de Nona probably treated many individuals with foot or leg problems and headaches, especially migraines.[46]

Dreams

From a medical perspective Hippocrates, Rufus of Ephesus (see Chapter 3) and Galen all acknowledged the importance of dreams. Galen recognised that some dreams were divine or prophetic such as those experienced in the *abaton*. Of the remainder, he sought to differentiate between those linked to a person's waking thoughts or actions – such as foods they had consumed – from dreams that were medically significant. The latter were said to reflect imbalances in an individual's humours (*dyskrasia*) (see Chapter 2). It was further believed that the soul could portray – through its visions – the humoral disturbances within the body. For example, if someone sees a destructive fire in a dream this was said to be due to an excess of yellow bile whereas a dream incorporating smoke, mist or darkness pointed to problems with black bile.[47]

Both the nature and the quantity of dreams were viewed by Hippocrates and Galen as being helpful in the diagnosis of a range of conditions. Moreover, in seeking to spot problems at an earlier stage Galen wrote:

> ... a dissimilarity to the previous pleasure in the actual food and drink taken is a sign of impending disease. So too is an unnatural blunting of thought processes, some unwonted forgetfulness, or sleep that is more troubled by dreams than before.[48]

110

Galen considered dreams another indicator of an individual's physical condition (see Chapter 3) and elaborated on the Hippocratic ideas by including factors outside of the dream in assessing their significance.

Dream analysis and interpretation were clearly important tools for Roman physicians to use in attempting to gain a better understanding of an individual's mind and psychological wellbeing. But Galen was always keen to use them only in conjunction with the traditional approaches of observing individuals, having conversations and speaking with friends and families.

What can the Romans teach us today?

Stoicism

Unlike our ancient forbears today's philosophical discissions are much more likely to be confined to universities than conducted in marketplaces, shopping centres, sports halls, theatres or restaurants. Few of us spend time seeking to discover a philosophy of life as opposed to striving for the latest consumer gadget, working to maximise our income or seeking to enhance our reputation and standing.

But, by writing this book during the period of the coronavirus pandemic in 2020, it became clear that some of the ideas developed by our Roman forbears have continuing relevance. The sales of *Meditations* rose dramatically during the year and, of particular interest, is the comment Marcus Aurelius made concerning the Antonine Plague that was ravaging the Empire at the time he was Emperor:

> *Infection of the mind is a far more dangerous pestilence than any unwholesomeness or disorder in the atmosphere around us. In so far as we are animals, the one attacks our lives; but as men, the other attacks our manhood.*[49]

In this, he was emphasising that it is not only plagues that matter but also our response to such crises based on our own thoughts and beliefs.

The Stoics pointed to two principal sources of human unhappiness that disturb our psychological wellbeing: a tendency to worry about things beyond our control and our insatiability. Much of the psychological damage linked to coronavirus has been generated more by our reactions to the outbreak than from the disease itself. Marcus Aurelius would remind us that it is important to distinguish between what we can control in our lives and what we cannot. This is about accepting that our plans can easily be thwarted by events beyond our control and to focus more on those things that are within our power to change, particularly our own judgements of events and our emotional state. None of us have any control over things such as natural events or disasters and we only have partial control over many other matters such as winning a match, getting a book published or securing a promotion. Stress, anxiety and depression are the consequences of worrying unduly about things over which we don't have complete control. However, we do have control over the goals we set for ourselves, the things we value, our character as well as the way we respond to comments from others. Admittedly, our goals might be frustrated by things beyond our control, but it is the setting of goals that matters as opposed to the precise outcomes.[50]

Marcus Aurelius argued that the key to having a good life and to prevent us 'misliving' is to learn to value things that are genuinely valuable and to be indifferent to things that lack value. He noted how the individuals he most admired lived in accordance with reason and exhibited the cardinal virtues of wisdom, justice, fortitude/courage and temperance/moderation.[51] According to Robertson, in determining our own values it is helpful to consider the following questions:[52]

- What is, ultimately, the most important thing in life to you?
- What do you really want your life to stand for or represent?
- What do you want to be remembered for after you are dead?
- What sort of person do you most want to be in life?
- What sort of character to you want to have?
- What do you want written on your tombstone?

Reason allows us to step back and to consider the consequences of our actions both for ourselves and for others. Linked to this is a recognition that we have many irrational desires and emotions such as fear, anger, craving, seeking fame and certain forms of pleasure that are bad for us and need to be replaced by healthy ones. Shakespeare is certainly highlighting this issue when Hamlet exclaims: '*Why, then, 'tis none to you, for there is nothing either good or bad, but thinking makes it so.*'[53]

The Stoics would advise that if something bad happens to us we need to avoid the use of emotive rhetoric or strong value judgements. We should strive to view events objectively and describe them in plain and simple terms, separating value judgements from facts. Losing a job is bad but, by focusing on the worst possible outcome, we can easily turn it into a catastrophe.

Galen, Seneca, Marcus Aurelius and Epictetus encouraged people to undertake morning and evening meditation, combined with mindfulness throughout the day.[54] One particularly important aspect of this is the anticipation of negative experiences that might be encountered and to build some emotional resilience. Meditation also provides an opportunity to practise negative visualisation. This means valuing and appreciating the things we already have – such as a house, a partner, a job, a life – and imagining the effect of their loss rather than constantly seeking for more 'things' such as possessions, fame or positive opinions of ourselves by others. In addition, it is about developing an awareness that bad things can and will happen but to keep a sense of perspective about what really matters.[55]

There is a clear link between modern cognitive behaviour therapy (CBT) and the writings of Epictetus and Marcus Aurelius. Both Aaron Beck and Albert Ellis, often regarded as the main pioneers of CBT, have stressed the role of Stoicism as a philosophical precursor of their respective approaches.[56] For example, the concept of radically accepting unpleasant feelings has been central to modern CBT – termed Stoic acceptance by the likes of Epictetus.[57] It is often easier to bear chronic pain by adopting the following Stoic principles:[58]

- Reminding ourselves that it is not the pain that upsets us but our judgement about the pain (cognitive distancing to CBT practitioners).
- Appreciating that the fear of pain does more harm than the pain itself (functional analysis to CBT practitioners).
- Viewing body sensations objectively rather than describing them in emotive terms (objective representation to CBT practitioners).

Healing sanctuaries

Inscriptions from Roman Africa in addition to the coins issued after the Antonine Plague suggest a resurgence of interest in Aesculapius and other healing deities, especially during the reigns of Caracalla and Septimius Severus.[59] The sanctuary of Nodens at Lydney was also probably founded during this same period.[60] It might be that various political and economic uncertainties from the latter half of the second century onwards – an 'age of anxiety' according to Dodds[61] – contributed to the appeal of such places.

From the large number of inscriptions and votives left by individuals in the sanctuaries at Epidaurus, Corinth and Athens, it seems likely that many benefited from visiting. The types of conditions where successful treatments are most-often mentioned were for people with chronic wounds, sores or skin problems; eye diseases including unilateral blindness; limb disorders such as paralysis or being lame; and infertility.[62] There was also a view that healing sanctuaries were the place to seek help for longstanding or intractable health problems. For example, Caelius Aurelianus specifically remarked that Aesculapius was *'the first to overcome diseases that are hard to heal'*.[63] Galen recalled seeing Aelius Aristides during one of his long periods of residence at the shrine in Pergamon and marvelled how such an obviously enfeebled body could be kept alive for a long while by his mental strength and will power.[64] Amazingly, Aelius Aristides also survived after catching the plague (probably smallpox) during the reign of Marcus Aurelius.

As discussed earlier, there is evidence that some surgical procedures were undertaken at healing sites such as draining abscesses or removing foreign bodies and that effective medicines such as opium were readily available. Particularly during the Roman period, it is suggested there was a gradual shift to more secular healing alongside the ritual supplications, with extended periods of residence at the healing sites and the employment of more individuals with medical or surgical skills.

Licking by snakes was also a key part of the treatment regimen in some situations and it now seems that snake saliva might have healing properties. Epidermal growth factor, a substance that stimulates a number of biological functions related to wound healing such as cell growth and the development of new blood vessels, was found to be present in the saliva of *Zamenis longissimus,* the species of snake associated with Aesculapian healing sanctuaries.[65]

Restoring tranquillity and psychological healing were probably facilitated by three key elements of healing sites – the choice of the location, the emphasis on locomotion and immersion in a broad range of psychological therapies.

Location

There can be little doubt that the locations for the numerous ancient healing sites found throughout the Greco-Roman world were very carefully selected to enhance wellbeing with trees, vistas, sunshine and fresh air. According to the Roman architect Vitruvius

for all temples there shall be chosen the most healthy sites with suitable springs in those places in which shrines are to be set up ... especially for Aesculapius and Salus and generally for those gods by whose medical power sick persons are manifestly healed. For when sick persons are moved from a pestilent to a healthy place and the water supply is from wholesome fountains, they will more quickly recover.[66]

Many ancient writers specifically commented on the locations and the surroundings of healing sanctuaries. For example, after visiting the temples at Canopus in Egypt, the Roman historian Ammianus Marcellinus wrote:

At a distance of twelve miles from Alexandria is Canopus ... The place is most delightful because of its beautiful pleasure-resorts, its soft air and healthful climate, so that anyone staying in that region believes that he is living outside of this world, as oftentimes he hears the winds that murmur a welcome with sunny breath.[67]

Even today, many ancient healing sites are places where it is possible to enjoy sunshine, breathe in cool clean air and to admire a view of the sea, a river or a stunning landscape. Visitors to Epidaurus are frequently struck by the open vistas, pure air and natural forest scents. The nearby Roman site at Corinth is often hot, dusty and affords little shelter, but by walking north for half a mile to reach the remains of the temple of Aesculapius, the environment becomes dramatically different. On the day I visited, a gentle cooling breeze was flowing up from the sea below and the outlook across the Gulf of Corinth and towards the distant hills beyond was magnificent [Plate 33].[68]

It is tempting to speculate that healing sites were chosen in accordance with the four ancient elements of fire, air, earth and water that also gave birth to the humoral theories (see Chapter 2). Nowadays, there is certainly a growing appreciation of the importance of the environment for good health and healing in terms of sunshine (perhaps linked to the ancient element of 'fire'), pure air, the sights and sounds of water in addition to landscape and contact with nature (perhaps linked to the ancient element of 'earth'). Getting outside into natural light will help to boost vitamin D levels and being among trees has been demonstrated to enhance both our wellbeing and immunity – known in Japan as *shinrin yoku* (forest bathing).[69]

Locomotion

Encouraging and facilitating movement was a particularly important aspect of the therapy delivered at healing sites (see Chapter 2). Reflecting on his time at the sanctuary in Pergamon, Aelius Aristides wrote: '*We were ordered to do many paradoxical things; among those that I recall there is a race which I had to run barefoot in winter-time, and again horse riding.*'[70] In addition, an inscription left by Marcus Apellas details the various exercises he undertook while at Epidaurus: running, walking (both with and without shoes), swinging on a swing, and rubbing against a wall.[71]

However, in addition to engaging in specific exercises, locomotion was about travelling to and from the site, moving around the sanctuary (often in a specific direction) and participating in various activities such as ceremonies, games, processions and festivals. Exercise would have been undertaken individually as well as with others in a group.

There is epigraphic evidence of visits to the healing site at Bath from several places across Britain: Caerleon, Cirencester, Chester, Lincoln and Gloucester. Dedicatory altars were also placed in the sanctuary by individuals originating from tribes around Trier and Chartres.[72] In journeying to Epidaurus, Marcus Apellas travelled by boat from his home at Mylasa (Turkey) via the Island of Aegina to Palaia Epidaurus. Following this, he then had to cover another ten kilometres overland – along the Sacred Way – before reaching the Aesculapian site.[73] Aelius Aristides set off with a spring in his step on his journey from his home to the rural sanctuary of Aesculapius at Poemanenos and to the warm springs of the Aesepus, writing: '*Then we started our journey, as if on pilgrimage, with cheerfulness, because the weather was wonderful and the road inviting.*'[74] On this occasion, he walked 30 kilometres (with around 11 kilometres being undertaken at night by torchlight).

There would also have been pilgrimages between healing sites and Aelius Aristides comments about his visits to a number of Aesculapia including Pergamon, Epidaurus and Smyrna.[75] The Emperor Caracalla travelled around various sanctuaries seeking help from Apollo Grannus, Aesculapius and Serapis with

> *many supplications and unwearying persistence. For even while abroad he sent to them prayers, sacrifices and votive offerings, and many couriers ran hither and thither every day carrying something of this kind; and he also went to them himself, hoping to prevail by appearing in person.*[76]

Some sanctuaries might even have been established in reasonably close proximity, perhaps encouraged by geographical or geological factors, in order to facilitate travel between them. Certainly, several potential healing sites have been identified around Trier in Germany[77] and along the Severn corridor in the UK.[78] North-west of the Severn were the sanctuaries at Lydney and Littledean and, across the water, is Bath in addition to possible healing sites at Great Whitcombe, Chedworth, Keynsham, Nettleton Scrub and Box.[79] It also seems likely that crossing the River Severn by ferry or ford was quite feasible for pilgrims during the Roman period.[80] The guest houses found at many sites, including Lydney, perhaps reflect the need for accommodation by travelling pilgrims. The example at Epidaurus contained at least 160 rooms and might even have had two floors.[81]

Visitors would have been encouraged to arrive at the major healing sanctuaries by following a particular route and using a specific entrance. The approach to the Aesculapian sanctuary at Pergamon was via an immense covered walkway, a colonnaded street, a covered passage and a forecourt prior to reaching the *propylaea* (monumental gateway). During this short journey individuals would have had their senses assailed by the sights of sculptures, water features and inscribed plaques; the sounds of vendors and of a busy city; and the smells of incense and medicinal herbs. The cacophony would then have faded as the pilgrims reached the forecourt; perhaps allowing them time and space to stop and view the sights ahead of them.[82]

The entry into the sanctuary at Epidaurus was also by means of a *propylaea*, located at the end of two wide highways, one from Epidaurus, the other from Argos [Plate 34]. It was both the point of arrival and a symbolic entrance into the sanctuary precinct, which was not enclosed with a wall but only surrounded by boundary stones. In addition to representing a transition into the sacred space, the *propylaea* was the first thing the pilgrims, as visitors or worshippers, would have encountered after their long journey to Epidaurus. The interior of the *propylaea* was divided into three aisles, the central one being the widest, and benches against the side walls provided visitors with an opportunity to rest and pause and to look over the sanctuary area before progressing onwards.[83]

Once inside the sanctuary, it seems likely that pilgrims were encouraged to follow a specific trail during which they could take in the sights, sounds and smells of the sanctuary in a specific order. Walking barefoot and touching objects as they passed might have also added a tactile sense to the experience. In addition, their route would have probably involved jostling with priests, officials, the infirm (and, perhaps, their concerned relatives), all going about their daily business, seeking treatment or making supplications to the gods.[84]

A careful analysis of the architecture at Pergamon suggests that the sanctuary was designed to facilitate movement as well as encouraging occasional slowing down (e.g. by the narrowing of passages or the need for climbing). This would have let individuals contemplate their surroundings in addition to pausing to admire the architecture, statuary and epigraphy.[85] During a promenade around Epidaurus, visitors would have encountered the inscription *'Pure must be he who enters the fragrant temple; purity means to think nothing but holy thoughts'*,[86] and, at Lambaesis the words *'Bonus intra, melior exi' ... enter a good man, leave a better one*.[87] Pilgrims could also have examined the testimonials left by individuals detailing portentous dreams and successful cures alongside a range of health-related votive offerings.

There seems little doubt that an expectant pilgrimage combined with immersion in the sights, sounds, smells and feel of a healing sanctuary would have had powerful psychological effects. Interestingly, it has recently been discovered that consciously watching for small wonders in the world around us during an otherwise ordinary walk can amplify the mental health benefits of a stroll, according to a psychological evaluation of what are termed 'awe walks'.[88]

Psychological therapies

From the moment that an individual set off for a healing site, they would have been subjected to a raft of psychological interventions designed to restore their tranquillity: group therapy, talking therapy, various arts therapies, dream healing; all combined with rest and relaxation. As discussed in the previous sub-sections, there was also an emphasis on locotherapy – the psychological benefits of locomotion as well as being in a specific place (location).

Inspiring confidence with the expectation of a positive outcome remains a key element of any treatment and this is more than simply a placebo effect.[89] The ancient healing sites seem to have been specifically designed to bolster a person's belief that a treatment will work and that they will get better. Also, the rapid cures of conditions such as unilateral blindness, mutism, paralysis or chronic headaches suggest the resolution of some underlying psychological disturbances. Galen noted the power of healing sites in instilling confidence in patients when he wrote:

Thus at any rate even among ourselves in Pergamum we see that those who are being treated by the god obey him when on many occasions he bids them not to drink at all for fifteen days, while they obey none of the physicians who give this prescription. For it has great influence on the patient's doing all which is prescribed if he has been firmly persuaded that a remarkable benefit to himself will ensue.[90]

Some of the specific treatments available at the various healing sites are certainly showing value today. For example, there is significant evidence for the effectiveness or music therapy in individuals with anxiety, depression, autism and dementia. For people living with cancer music may have beneficial effects on anxiety, pain, fatigue, depression, and quality of life. Drama, painting and drawing have also been used to promote mental health; and bibliotherapy – often combined with writing therapy – has been shown to be effective in the treatment of depression. Bibliotherapy involves storytelling or the reading of specific texts with the purpose of healing. It uses an individual's relationship to the content of books and poetry and other written words as therapy.[91]

Aesculapian temple medicine is mysterious – and foreign – to many doctors today, mixing traditional practices such as surgery and pharmacology with magic and ritual. Although I might feel comfortable with enhancing wellbeing by encouraging people to exercise, eat sensibly and bathe – 'dream healing' is not something I have yet to recommend. However, during the coronavirus outbreak some individuals have been psychologically traumatised by their experiences and many people have reported disturbing dreams and nightmares. By not asking patients about their dreams, doctors might be ignoring some important diagnostic information and, as suggested by Galen, an opportunity to spot some conditions earlier. Also, from a psychological perspective, both Freud and Jung believed that dreams are worth examining as they might represent unconscious wishes or unrecognised information. More recently, it has been suggested that dreams help us to process emotions – especially negative ones.[92]

Prior to the advent of coronavirus individuals such as Dr Edward Tick had been arranging 'dream healing' pilgrimages to the Aesculapian sites in Greece to try to help people – especially war veterans – overcome specific psychological problems. In addition to encouraging and interpreting a person's dreams, other key elements of the approach include immersion in the archaeology, the history, the thoughts and the words of our classical forbears.[93]

Today, there is little doubt that coronavirus has inflicted, and will continue to inflict, significant psychological damage on the population. Also, we will need to recognise that there is much more to recovering from a plague than just medicines, scans and outpatient visits. Natural disasters make us look at things afresh and this might involve challenging some of our modern assumptions and priorities with a greater focus on whole patient care, including the potential role of healing sanctuaries. There is certainly already some evidence for the health benefits of week-long, holistic, multifaceted, residential retreats.[94]

CHAPTER 7

Surgical and Physical Therapies

A wide range of surgical procedures in addition to a number of physical therapies were available to Roman patients. Celsus described more than one hundred operations including amputations, open abdominal surgery and the couching of cataracts; in addition to cupping, massaging and bathing.[1] The physician Asclepiades of Bithynia was a particular advocate of rubbing, the use of rocking applies and various hydrotherapies.[2]

Surgery

There are several stone-carved representations of surgical instrument collections on Roman funerary monuments and a wall painting from Pompeii of a wounded Aeneas, clearly illustrates the removal of an arrowhead using forceps [Plate 5]. Also, by the early years of the first century AD, an increasingly large number of distinctive, purpose-made, metal tools labelled as 'surgical' begin to appear in the archaeological record from military, civilian and religious sites.[3] Their identification often rests on comparisons being made with descriptions contained in classical medical texts. In 1907, Milne assembled an extensive inventory of Greek and Roman surgical instruments that he grouped into knives, probes and hooks, forceps, cautery tools, needles and cannulas; in addition to bone, dental, bladder and gynaecological instruments.[4]

However, although we might have a view about the role of a particular object in relation to both modern and ancient surgical practice, whether it really served that purpose can sometimes be debatable. Today's doctors clearly perform a different spectrum of operations using some dissimilar surgical techniques than did their

Roman predecessors. Moreover, some of the injuries sustained during battle in the ancient world would have been quite distinct from those encountered in modern warfare and obviously required different approaches. The absence of effective anaesthesia would have also been an important consideration for the Roman surgeon. Celsus wrote that:

if it is a broad weapon which has been embedded, it is not expedient to extract it through a counter opening, lest we add a second large wound to one already large. It is therefore to be pulled out by the aid of some such instrument as that which the Greeks call the Dioclean cyathiscus.[5]

Majno suggests that this was a spoon-shaped object with a small hole at the base to take the point of a spear or arrowhead. It would have been passed down into the wound and then rotated slightly to accommodate the weapon, which could have then been withdrawn.[6]

The repair of a simple flesh wound was the most commonly performed surgical procedure in the ancient world. It would have been undertaken by doctors but also a range of other individuals, such as a family member or, in the case of the army, a fellow soldier.[7] Basic surgical kits consisting of probes, hooks, forceps, needles, cautery tools and scalpels were certainly readily available [Plate 35].[8] Such instruments have been found scattered widely across Pompeii indicating that, perhaps, minor surgical procedures could have been performed in a variety of locations including homes and bathhouses (see also Chapter 4).[9]

Celsus explained that:

if the wound is in a soft part, it should be stitched up, and particularly when the cut is in the tip of the ear or the point of the nose or forehead or cheek or eyelid or lip or the skin over the throat or abdomen. But if the wound is in the flesh, and gapes, and its margins are not easily drawn together, then stitching is

*unsuitable; fibulae (the Greeks call them ancteres) are then to
be inserted, which draw together the margins to some extent and
so render the subsequent scar less broad.*[10]

Stitching with a needle and thread was not dissimilar to the approach
used today, perhaps using curved needles made of bone or metal.
However, effecting a closure with *fibulae* might have entailed passing
copper-alloy skewers through the wound [Plate 36]. Subsequently,
threads would have been looped around the skewers in a figure-of-eight
fashion while the surgeon squeezed the edges of the wound together.[11]

In the absence of antibiotics, the use of *fibulae* may have been
particularly appropriate in situations where there were concerns about
inflammation or infection and Celsus explained that '*fibulae leave the
wound wider open … in order that there may be an outlet for any
humour collecting within*'.[12] John Ratcliffe also argues that *fibulae*
would stabilise the wound, the copper ions released from the skewers
would have had anti-bacterial effects and, should there be any swelling,
the threads could have been adjusted.[13]

Celsus described two approaches to dealing with varicose veins;
using cautery or by excision writing that in:

*the method of cauterisation: the overlying skin is incised, then
the exposed vein is pressed upon moderately with a fine, blunt,
hot cautery iron, avoiding a burn of the margins of the incision,
which can easily be done by retracting them with hooks.*[14]

Such skin hooks are relatively common archaeological finds, and, in
the absence of anaesthesia, they might have been much less painful
for patients in comparison with dissecting forceps.[15]

As ancient medicine was built on different theories and ideas than
is modern medical practice (see Chapter 2), some of the surgical
procedures described by Roman authors would, perhaps, be labelled
inappropriate or cosmetic today. Excision of the uvula was often

undertaken by Roman surgeons[16] but, in the UK, it is now rare; only occasionally being used as a component of an overall surgical approach to ameliorate snoring. However, uvulectomy by traditional practitioners in Africa is an age-long practice and still remains a common procedure in Nigeria.[17] Three sets of uvula forceps (*staphylagra*) have been unearthed in Britain and, as can be seen from the illustration of the Caerwent example, the branches of the forceps are crossed and pivot around a rivet joint like a pair of scissors [Plate 37]. This particular instrument is 19.4cm long and the jaws, which project forward enclosing a cup for the amputated uvula, bear fine teeth. The teeth were probably used to crush the neck of the uvula thereby reducing the chances of haemorrhage, which was quite a problem if the uvula was simply cut.[18] The Romans also viewed hair removal as an important approach to treating several diseases and shaving knives could thus be considered potential surgical tools as well as razors.[19]

Several possible surgical tools have been discovered in a grave dating from the AD 50s at Stanway near Colchester and, intriguingly, the more typical operative instruments (i.e. scalpels, hooks, forceps, needles and a saw) were accompanied by eight divination rods. It seems likely that these rods would have been cast on the ground and the resulting distribution read, perhaps for diagnostic or prognostic purposes. However, if the rods were an integral component of a patient's surgical care then, perhaps, they should be considered as medical instruments too.[20]

One of the major problems of some modern classifications of ancient tools is that they sometimes do not appreciate the generic nature of such objects. Hammers and chisels were used in cranial surgery but also by blacksmiths and carpenters (and, occasionally, by other healers to make splints for fractures). A number of clearly identifiable surgical instruments have been discovered at Wroxeter but whether the Roman lead hammer found there was surgical or otherwise can only be guessed at.[21] Even today, many of the instruments found in an orthopaedic surgeon's instrument tray would not be out of place in a cabinet maker's workshop – e.g. saws, bone levers, bone forceps and drills. Celsus highlighted this issue in his description of the replacement of a bone in a compound fracture:

> *when a small fragment of bone projects ... it is pushed back into place ... and if this cannot be done with the hand, pincers, such as smiths use, must be applied ... [and] force the projecting bone into place.*[22]

The blacksmiths tongs found at Tremadoc in Wales are most likely the type recommended by Celsus and might also have been 'surgical'.[23]

There is also evidence of treatment variations across the Roman Empire and Celsus stated that '*methods of practice differ according to the nature of localities, and that one method is required in Rome, another in Egypt, another in Gaul*'.[24] Thus, some tools may have been employed in a different fashion in Roman Britain than elsewhere, and it is possible that certain medical instruments being used in the provinces did not even warrant a mention in the elite Roman texts. In addition, and especially in the more peripheral regions of the Roman Empire, a surgical instrument may have been utilised for more than one purpose. For example, a *staphylagra* could have been enlisted to treat haemorrhoids in addition to problems relating to the uvula. Also, hybrid tools are not uncommon with different instruments being found at either end of a single handle. Combinations identified to date include: scalpel with blunt dissector, sharp hook with blunt hook, forceps with sharp hook, needle or probe, lithotomy knife and scoop, double blunt hook, double bone lever, double needle and double probe.[25]

Most Roman scalpels combined a robust copper-alloy handle, incorporating a grip and blunt dissector, with a fine and hard-edged, but less durable, iron blade. The blade was soldered into the handle, which was sometimes elaborately decorated.[26] Two main varieties of scalpels have been identified by Jackson: Type I has a deep-bellied iron blade, whereas Type II is slenderer, perhaps being used for more delicate work.[27] John Ratcliffe, a retired surgeon, tested the effectiveness of a Type I facsimile on a piece of pork belly and concluded that it was ideal for making rapid and deep incisions.[28]

Forceps had a key place in Roman surgery; they could be used for holding tissues, removing splints or eyelashes. However, the problem is that depilation was also a feature of civilisation as a hairless body was perceived as the Roman ideal. In determining whether a particular find had a surgical or a cosmetic/social role, it is now generally agreed that a forceps greater than 8cm long and of better craftsmanship is more likely to have had been used for operations.[29] The Littleborough forceps, for example, [Plate 38] was made in one piece from brass. It is 15.5cm long and consists of two elements: the forceps itself and a crook-shaped hook.[30] In common with a similar type of surgical forceps found at Silchester, it seems likely that a metal slider linked the arms together.[31] The jaws of the forceps are 17mm wide and, on each of the edges, serrations had been carefully cut such that the two jaws interlocked exactly. Of particular interest, and by analogy with an identical example from Trier, it has been suggested that the tip of the hook was stylised as a snake's head, representing a link between the user and Aesculapius (see Chapter 6).

In searching for the effects of ancient surgical practices in the archaeological record, it is important to appreciate that very few operations will leave any tangible palaeopathological evidence on surviving human remains. An undisplaced fracture will heal in exactly the same way as will a break in which bone forceps or bone elevators had been used to reposition the bones. However, Celsus described trephination for head wounds in which some bone was removed by a *modiolus 'a hollow cylindrical iron instrument with its lower edges serrated; in the middle of which is fixed a pin which is itself surrounded by an inner disc'.*[32] He then went on to explain that:

> *the pressure must be such that it both bores and rotates; for if pressed lightly it makes little advance, if heavily it does not*

rotate. It is a good plan to drop in a little rose oil or milk, so that it may rotate more smoothly; but if too much is used the keenness of the instrument is blunted. When a way has been cut by the modiolus, the central pin is taken out, and the modiolus worked by itself; then, when the bone dust shows that underlying bone is sound, the modiolus is laid aside.[33]

Two examples of *modioli* have been identified at Bingen as well as seven skulls exhibiting drilled trephinations at Guntramsdorf and Katzelsdorf.[34] Three likely examples of trephination have also been found in Britain: Whitchurch, York and Cirencester. In the latter example it seems that the skull might have been pressing on the brain, perhaps inducing fits. Moreover, the evidence of new bone growth around the area of the trephine suggests that this patient also survived the surgery.[35]

Jackson emphasises the importance of context in assigning a surgical role to a tool that could have had a variety of uses and, occasionally, sudden catastrophic events such as volcanic eruptions or fires will preserve collections of instruments in situ. A small set of instruments being carried by one of the victims of Vesuvius at Pompeii comprised four scalpels, two forceps, two hooks, six probes and two needles.[36] A building termed the '*Domus del chirurgo*' at Rimini was burnt down by the Alamani in AD 257–258 during their attack on Northern Italy, and then immediately backfilled to strengthen the neighbouring town wall. Excavations in 1989 brought to light 150 surgical instruments of a variety of types and designs.[37]

The Rimini set was a particularly exciting find as it appeared to represent a complete assemblage of surgical instruments within its original context. Over forty scalpels and surgical knives, nineteen spring forceps, a range of sharp and blunt hooks, surgical needles and probes have been identified. In addition, there were some forty instruments for bone surgery including two folding copper-alloy handles for operating trepans, solid-tipped drills, three sequestrum forceps for seizing and removing bone fragments, levers for elevating fractured bones, chisels, three gouges, four *lenticula* (guarded chisels), a finely toothed iron saw-knife and a small iron file. The file could also have been used in dentistry and the presence of seven iron forceps suggests dental practice too. Other specialist instruments included two *staphylagra* and an *uncus*, for performing lithotomy.[38]

Cataract extraction was well described by Celsus:

> *he is to be seated opposite the surgeon in a light room, facing the light, while the surgeon sits on a slightly higher seat; the assistant from behind holds the head so that the patient does not move: for vision can be destroyed permanently by a slight movement ... Thereupon a needle is to be taken pointed enough to penetrate, yet not too fine, and this is to be inserted straight through the two outer tunics at a spot intermediate between the pupil of the eye and the angle adjacent to the temple, away from the middle of the cataract, in such a way that no vein is wounded. The needle should not be, however, entered timidly ... When the [correct] spot is reached, the needle is to be sloped ... and should gently rotate there and little by little guide it [i.e. the lens with the cataract] below the region of the pupil.*[39]

Possible cataract needles have been found at Carlisle and Piddington and a copper-alloy probe case dredged from the bed of the river Saône contained three examples.[40] Most are sharpened at one end and angled with a small swelling at the other [Plate 39]. Once the cataract had been displaced perhaps the end metal blob was heated and then used for cauterising the wound.

Bathing and hydrotherapy

Nowadays, we might view baths simply in terms of cleanliness but, to the Romans, bathhouses were also about improving general health and wellbeing in addition to specific healing (see Chapter 4). Classical authors often recommended taking or avoiding baths, either hot or cold, not only as remedies for all sorts of ailments, but also for the preservation of health (see Chapter 2). Galen's writings are peppered with references to bathing for medical purposes and Celsus refers to baths 56 times in a remedial connection and 11 times in a preventive one.[41]

In accordance with humoral theory (see Chapter 2) bathing was viewed as a way of regulating the balance to '*draw out corrupt humour and change the bodily habit*',[42] by means of heating, cooling, moistening or drying. In addition, Celsus emphasised the importance of sweating in addressing humoral excesses writing: '*sweating also is elicited in two ways, either by dry heat, or by the bath*'.[43] He also went on to discuss the appropriate and careful use of baths for patients with fevers in addition to a variety of more specific problems such as headaches, worm infestations, boils and liver abscesses. In relation to fever, he viewed bathing as having two purposes: '*after fevers have been dissipated, it forms for a convalescent the preliminary to a fuller diet and stronger wine; at another time it actually takes off the fever*.'[44]

The physician Asclepiades of Bithynia was a great advocate of hydrotherapy, especially cold- treatments using a blanket-like material impregnated with water, termed a fomentation. He viewed the body as comprising units (*corpuscles*), which were separated by spaces or ducts (*pores*). The free movement of *corpuscles* was what kept a person healthy, but hindrance of their movement by over-widening or blocking of the *pores* caused illness. Should the *pores* be too wide, cold water would help to close them; should they be too narrow, sweating and hot water would assist in opening them. For Asclepiades, baths provided the perfect means to optimise the activities of the *pores* and *corpuscles*: hot or cold, dry or wet.[45]

Antonius Musa successfully adopted Asclepiades' cold-water application in the treatment of the Emperor Augustus. Suetonius wrote that:

> *when abscesses on the liver reduced him to such despair that*
> *he consented to try a remedy which ran counter to all medical*

practice: because hot fomentations afforded him no relief, his physician Antonius Musa successfully prescribed cold ones.[46]

One other specific water treatment suggested by Asclepiades were 'hanging baths' *pensiles balineae*[47] ... probably a form of hot bathing using tanks of heated water, perhaps even a type of shower?

Pliny the Elder devoted book 31 of his *Naturalis historia* to water and, in Chapter 2, he wrote about natural springs:

nowhere do they abound in greater number, or offer a greater variety of medicinal properties than in the Gulf of Baiae; some being impregnated with sulphur, some with alum, some with salt, some with nitre, and some with bitumen, while others are of a mixed quality, partly acid and partly salt. In other cases, again, it is by their vapours that waters are so beneficial to man.[48]

He then went on to discuss the use of specific waters – drunk, bathed in, or applied hot or cold – as remedies for infertility, urinary stones, wound healing, memory problems and male insanity. In terms of mechanisms of action, Vitruvius commented that:

sulphur springs refresh muscular weakness by heating and burning poisonous humours from the body. Alum springs affect parts of the body which are dissolved by paralysis or some stroke of disease; they warm through the open pores and overcome the cold by the opposing power of the heat, and thus forthwith the diseased parts are restored to their ancient health.[49]

Warm water bathing – heated naturally or artificially – was more generally recommended for a variety of conditions including joint and ligament problems, back pain, gout and digestive disorders. It was also suggested that warm baths helped to allow nutritious food to be assimilated.[50]

Massage and rocking

In an extensive discussion of massage in his second book on *Hygiene*, Galen considered it both a specific therapy as well as an adjunct to something else, especially exercise. He provided a detailed account of massage categorising it by quality (i.e. hard/firm, soft/gentle, moderate) and quantity (i.e. little, much, moderate).[51] More specifically, he wrote that:

> *in the preparatory massage before exercises, which has the objective of softening the bodies, it is necessary for a quality midway between hard and soft to prevail, and to model everything in relation to that. The rubbings should be of various kinds with laying on and moving around of the hands, not only moving them from above downward and from below upward, but also sideways, crosswise, obliquely and circularly.*[52]

Celsus echoed Hippocrates and Asclepiades in recommending massaging for a wide variety of conditions stating that '*rubbing, if strenuous, hardens the body, if gentle, relaxes; if much, it diminishes, if moderate, fills out*'.[53] For example, '*prolonged headaches are relieved by rubbing of the head, although not at the height of the pain*'.[54]

Rocking, another recommendation of Asclepiades, was seen as '*very suitable for chronic maladies which are already abating; it is also of service both for those who are now entirely free of fever, but cannot as yet themselves take exercise*'.[55] Celsus explained that:

> *the gentlest rocking is that on board ship either in harbour or in a river, more severe is that aboard ship on the high seas, or in a litter or even severer in a carriage: but each of these can be intensified or mitigated. Failing any of the above, the bed should be so slung as to be swayed.*[56]

Cupping and phlebotomy

Cupping is performed by applying cups to selected skin points and creating a sub-atmospheric pressure. In simple dry cupping, suction is used to draw the skin inside the vessel without any additions. Wet cupping is the application of a suction vessel after the skin has been cut in order to draw out blood.[57] Celsus wrote that:

> there are two kinds of cups, one made of bronze, the other of horn. The bronze cup is open at one end, closed at the other; the horn one, likewise at one end open, has at the other a small hole. Into the bronze cup is put burning lint, and in this state its mouth is applied and pressed to the body until it adheres. The horn cup is applied as it is to the body, and when the air is withdrawn by the mouth through the small hole at the end, and after the hole has been closed by applying wax over it, the horn cup likewise adheres.[58] [Plate 40]

To the Romans bloodletting (phlebotomy) using wet cupping or applying leaches was a means of balancing the humours by removing an excess of blood in those with *plethora*.[59] But, over his career, Galen became increasingly ambivalent about this treatment, eventually commenting that '*it is not the easiest thing to identify all who need the remedy, just as it is not easy to decide on the amount to be taken, or which vein to cut, or the time to do it*'.[60] He certainly never used it in children under the age of fourteen, the frail elderly or those with poor constitutions.

What can the Romans teach us today?

In relation to surgery, it could be argued that modern practitioners have much more that they could teach the Romans than vice versa! But, although today's surgeons will certainly deliver considerably better operative outcomes than their ancient forbears, very few are likely to be permitted to develop new tools or techniques and use them on their patients. There is also a shift in emphasis towards greater specialisation with the risk that some modern surgeons might not adequately consider alternative treatment approaches.

Physical therapies provided to my patients in NHS settings are also narrowly focused being generally confined to various versions of physiotherapy. Twenty-five years ago, a former chief medical officer even remarked to me that the true indicator of an effective health service in relation to physical treatments was one that, based on the research evidence, spent more money on alternatives such as osteopathy and less on physiotherapy.[61]

Technical responsibility

Galen was very particular about the instruments he used for surgery, remarking that the best quality of steel for manufacture was sourced from Noricum.[62] After a fire in Rome, he wrote how it had destroyed:

instruments of every kind. Some, valuable for medical purposes, I said I had lost but still hoped to replace, but that other instruments I had invented myself, making models out of wax before handing them over to the bronze-smiths, these I cannot replace without a great deal of time and effort.[63]

Echoing his approach to pharmaceuticals (see Chapter 5), Galen was clearly intimately involved in the design and development of his surgical tools.

Several authors have highlighted the extraordinary craftsmanship, design, décor and ingenuity of many Roman medical instruments.[64] For some isolated finds – such as the Hockwold uterine sound – their technical and aesthetic characteristics have played a significant part in helping to categorise them as medical.[65] Ratcliffe specifically comments on the remarkable skill that would have been required to make the very thin needle, of the order of 300–500 microns in diameter, to carry a human hair as described by Celsus.[66]

To better understand the technicalities underpinning the manufacture of a particularly complex piece of Roman medical equipment, I persuaded Martin Jones, a semi-retired Design Technology teacher, to work with me to make a facsimile of a Roman eye medicine box. In 1990, Boyer had described the excavation of a cremation burial from Lyon in which was found a brass box with four compartments that contained twenty baton-shaped collyria (see Chapter 5).[67] Using Boyer's description, together with a very useful video of the preservation of the Lyon box available on-line,[68] Martin Jones produced a beautiful copy [Plates 41 and 42].

The dimensions of the box are length 114mm, width 65mm and height 28mm. In keeping with the original, it consists of thirteen individual pieces of brass sheet (0.56mm thick) joined together by soft solder. Inside the box are five small compartments covered by a sliding lid held in place by a tongue-shaped locking mechanism. On the underside is a cup-shaped depression in the brass – spherical diameter 42.5mm, depth 13.7mm.

Four particularly challenging elements of the reconstruction were selecting an appropriate solder (and soldering approach), making the cup-shaped hollow, fitting in the lid for the central compartment and understanding the locking mechanism. The difficulty with the soldering was to produce a resilient box – suitable for a travelling eye healer – without melting any previously soldered joints or the brass itself. The original plan was to use a hard silver solder for the basic box structure and then to add in the other components using a lower temperature soft solder. But initial experiments with silver solder proved to be very difficult due to the high melting temperature combined with the thin brass being used. As a result, several parts had to be re-made because of damage to the brass. The final construction using soft solder with heat sinks worked much better than had originally been anticipated.

To produce the cup-shaped depression, a series of hardwood punches and formers had to be made and then, with regular annealing, the brass sheet was gradually beaten to the shape and depth required. Meanwhile, the remainder of the brass sheet had to be carefully clamped in place to prevent any distortion of the surrounding areas. Fitting the lids onto the compartments (on pin hinges) proved to be reasonably straightforward until the central compartment was attempted. This presented another challenge and explained why the manufacturer of the Lyon box had inserted small pieces of steel to allow springing of the opposing walls. This permitted the central lid to be positioned in place while the walls were momentarily held out of position. This reconstruction highlights the extraordinary technical skills of the Romans.

The completed box would have been opened by pressing the central springing button allowing the tongue-shaped swivel to rotate anti-clockwise. The bevelled brass lid could then be retracted revealing five lidded brass compartments containing a range of embossed collyria. The peripatetic eye healer would have selected and removed a collyrium from inside the box and cut off a small piece. The residue then being put back into the relevant compartment and the box secured again with the sliding lid. After crushing the collyrium fragment on a stone palate using a brass probe, the resulting powder would have been mixed with water, egg or milk as appropriate in the cup-shaped depression on the underside of the box to produce a paste for application to the eye (see Chapter 5).

There seems little doubt that Roman smiths and doctors worked together to produce some stunning and technically challenging tools. Subsequently, in the nineteenth century and the first decades of the twentieth century, there was a similar explosion of new surgical instruments combined with the development of numerous innovative surgical procedures. New materials, such as stainless steel, chrome, titanium and vanadium were then also available for the manufacturing of such instruments. But, more recently, increasingly strict regulatory controls have both constrained and modified the ancient path of innovation (see also Chapter 3).[69]

However, irrespective of the quality or the glitter of the surgical instruments being used in any era, it is always worth bearing in mind the remark by the second-century satirist Lucian:

You are similar to the fake physicians who buy themselves silver cupping-glasses, lancets with gold handles, all encased in ivory. But they do not know how to use the tools when the time comes and make way for a proper doctor who produces a knife with a sharp edge but which has a rusty handle.[70]

Both Galen and Celsus also emphasised the importance of a sound grounding in anatomy. In seeking out the best surgeon, the prospective patient is advised, according to Galen, first to *'find out how wide his knowledge is and how penetrative is his training in anatomy'*.[71]

The appropriate use of surgery

Based on a detailed assessment of some of the operations described by Celsus, Ratcliffe concluded that *'his surgery, when judged in the light of modern practice was reasoned, skilled and highly appropriate for contemporary circumstances'*.[72] The Romans also adopted a particularly measured approach to undertaking surgery, always considering alternative approaches such as hygiene or pharmaceuticals (see Chapters 2 and 5). Major surgical procedures were a last resort for the ancients, being fraught with dangers of infection or permanent disability, aside from the considerable pain that must have been experienced in the absence of any effective anaesthetic techniques.[73]

Celsus specifically commented on the indications as well as the contra-indications for a variety of surgical techniques. For example, he wrote *'if the uvula, owing to inflammation is elongated downwards, and is painful and dusky red in colour, it cannot be cut away without danger'*.[74] He also outlined the four key signs of inflammation (redness and swelling with heat and pain) that still apply in assessing wounds, including those made by surgeons. Celsus exact words were *'notae vero inflammationis sunt quattuor: rubor et tumor cum calore et dolore'*.[75]

Few surgeons would take issue with Galen in his recognition of the importance of undertaking sufficient operations to ensure that expertise is maintained, producing the best outcomes for patients. He commented that he would have performed a particular surgical treatment *'if I had remained throughout in Asia. However, as I have spent most of my time in Rome, I have followed the custom of the city, yielding the majority of such activities to those they call surgeons'*.[76]

Recent developments in numerous aspects of surgery, anaesthesia and infection control have, perhaps, encouraged some modern surgeons to operate when alternatives might be considered. For example, particular concerns have been raised about the inappropriate use of some gynaecological procedures in addition to gall bladder surgery.[77] This century has also seen the growth in a movement termed 'choosing wisely' specifically designed to root out ineffective or inappropriate surgical procedures.[78]

Physical therapies

There is a growing body of modern research evidence in favour of bathing, hydrotherapy and balneotherapy (bathing in spa water).[79] For example, aquatic exercise reduces pain and disability in addition to improving quality of life for individuals with osteoarthritis in the knee or hip.[80] Both hot water bathing and sauna bathing seem to have beneficial effects in reducing various risk factors for heart and circulatory diseases.[81]

Massage therapy also appears to be effective in ameliorating pain and improving health-related quality of life for a variety of health conditions.[82] In a study of back problems, massage was found to be helpful irrespective of whether it was designed to manipulate soft tissues or to bring about relaxation.[83] For knee osteoarthritis a sixty-minute once weekly dose of massage has been recommended by some.[84]

Therapeutic rocking or cupping are not things that I have ever suggested to any patient. But there is now some evidence for the health benefits of rocking chair therapy in individuals with dementia or substance misuse.[85] However, despite its popularity in some quarters, more rigorous studies are required before the effectiveness of cupping for the treatment of pain can be determined.[86] Today, phlebotomy therapy is restricted to a few conditions such as haemochromatosis or polycythaemia and may have a place for some individuals with metabolic syndrome.[87] Galen's caution around cupping and bloodletting still appears very well-founded.

CHAPTER 8

Conclusion

Three hundred years ago, Christian Gruner wrote:

For in the monuments of the ancients there are the seeds and principles of manifold and various doctrine, and it is very important to know what and how much they have written about medical affairs, what decrees and precepts they have left consigned to their successors, either for imitation, or for condemnation, or for restraint.[1]

From the care of individuals to the protection of the wellbeing of populations the Romans undoubtedly bequeathed us a substantial legacy. Within this book I have explored ancient technical and hygienic achievements and considered the place of healers in Roman society, in addition to looking at the effectiveness of their approaches to both preventing and treating a range of physical and psychological problems.

Although Greco-Roman medicine was a dominant force well into the Middle Ages, it began to fall from favour by the sixteenth century. In the 1540s, Andreas Vesalius identified several errors in Galen's work on human anatomy due to an over-reliance on animal dissection. Subsequently, Harvey's discovery of the circulation of the blood raised questions about the Greco-Roman understanding of physiology. In addition, some of the ancient treatments began to be viewed as outdated, eccentric or, on occasions, downright dangerous. Gradually, the writings of individuals such as Galen, Celsus and Scribonius Largus migrated away from medical faculties, finding a new home in departments of philology. The interest was no longer in the relevance of the classical texts for health and wellbeing, but rather around issues such as authenticity, translation and word definition.

However, I would contend that great wisdom can be found buried in the ancient sources that might still assist with many of today's health concerns and dilemmas. As discussed in Chapter 2, Galen's focus on access to fresh air, movement, sensible eating and getting sufficient sleep matter as much today as they did in the past. Our forebears can also help us to determine the best balances between prevention and treatment, centralised control and individual responsibility, as well as the most appropriate use of technology, drugs and surgery.

Trust between patients and their carers remains the cornerstone of good health care and, echoing Scribonius Largus' comments in Chapter 3, there is an urgent requirement to reemphasise the importance of humanity over regulation. Also, as discussed in Chapter 5, modern research indicates that ancient compound pharmaceutical remedies are worthy of further examination. Chapter 6 outlines several different approaches to enhancing psychological wellbeing and restoring tranquillity including Stoicism, locotherapy and dream healing that could have value for numerous individuals trying to cope with the stresses and strains of modern life.

But there are also some aspects of the classical medical past that we should be very cautious about mimicking such as cupping, purging and the deification of health care institutions. As was the case for Aesculapius and Apollo, the NHS is now being commemorated on coins, inscriptions, and, even, at religious services and the London Olympics. During the course of the coronavirus pandemic, votive images have appeared in many house windows, combined with widespread encouragement to applaud the NHS at a fixed time each week.

The medical voices and ideas from the Greco-Romans do still have relevance today but, in addition, we have access to a specific therapy by immersing ourselves in the remains they have left behind.[2] Helping to run a coronavirus-secure excavation at Roman Brough (*Petuaria*), getting involved in developing a Roman garden at Aldborough and leading a walk around the Roman camps at Cawthorn during the summer of 2020 certainly confirmed to me the enormous benefits of such activities in enhancing people's physical and psychological wellbeing.

APPENDIX 1

The Hippocratic Oath
(tr, WHS Jones, 1923)

I swear by Apollo Physician, by Aesculapius, by Health, by Panacea, and by all the gods and goddesses, making them my witnesses, that I will carry out, according to my ability and judgment, this oath and this indenture.

To hold my teacher in this art equal to my own parents; to make him partner in my livelihood; when he is in need of money to share mine with him; to consider his family as my own brothers, and to teach them this art, if they want to learn it, without fee or indenture; to impart precept, oral instruction, and all other instruction to my own sons, the sons of my teacher, and to indentured pupils who have taken the physician's oath, but to nobody else.

I will use treatment to help the sick according to my ability and judgment, but never with a view to injury and wrongdoing. Neither will I administer a poison to anybody when asked to do so, nor will I suggest such a course. Similarly I will not give to a woman a pessary to cause abortion. But I will keep pure and holy both my life and my art. I will not use the knife, not even, verily, on sufferers from stone, but I will give place to such as are craftsmen therein.

Into whatsoever houses I enter, I will enter to help the sick, and I will abstain from all intentional wrong-doing and harm, especially from abusing the bodies of man or woman, bond or free. And whatsoever I shall see or hear in the course of my profession, as well as outside my profession in my intercourse with men, if it be what should not be published abroad, I will never divulge, holding such things to be holy secrets.

Now if I carry out this oath, and break it not, may I gain for ever reputation among all men for my life and for my art; but if I transgress it and forswear myself, may the opposite befall me.

Titles and Translations of Greek and Roman Literary Sources

Author and title	English title	Edition and translation
Ammianus Marcellinus *Res Gestae*	*The Roman History of Ammianus Marcellinus*	Wallace-Hadrill (1986)
Aelius Aristides *Hieroi Logoi*	*Sacred Tales*	Behr (1981 and 1986)
Aelius Aristides *Orationes*	*Orations*	Behr (1981 and 1986)
Cato *De agri cultura*	*On Agriculture*	Hooper and Ash (1935)
Celsus *De medicina*	*On Medicine*	Spencer (1971)
Columella *De re rustica*	*On Agriculture*	Ash (1941)
Dio Cassius *Historia Romana*	*Roman History*	Foster (1914)
Dioscorides *De materia medica*	*On Medical Material*	Beck (2005)
Epictetus *Encheiridion*	*Handbook of Epictetus*	Long (2018)
Frontinus *De aquis urbis Romae*	*The Aqueducts of Rome*	Bennett (1925)
Fronto *Epistulae ad Marcum Caesarem*	*Letters to Marcus Aurelius*	Haines (1919)
Galen *De alimentorum facultatibus*	*On the Properties of Foodstuffs*	Powell (2003)

Author and title	English title	Edition and translation
Galen *Ars medica*	*The Art of Medicine*	Johnston (2016)
Galen *De constitutione artis medicae*	*On the Constitution of the Art of Medicine*	Johnston (2016)
Galen *De causis morborum*	*On the Causes of Diseases*	Johnston (2006)
Galen *De causis symptomatum*	*On the Causes of Symptoms*	Johnston (2006)
Galen *De libris propriis*	*My Own Books*	Singer (1997)
Galen *De locis affectis*	*On the Affected Parts*	Siegel (1976)
Galen *De methodo medendi*	*The Method of Medicine*	Johnston and Horsley (2011)
Galen *Quod optimus medicus sit quoque philosophus*	*The Best Doctor Is also a Philosopher*	Singer (1997)
Galen *De parvae pilae exercitio*	*On Exercise with the Small Ball*	Johnston (2018)
Galen *De praecognitione [ad Epigenem]*	*On Prognosis [for Epigenes]*	Nutton (1979)
Galen *De ptisana*	*On Barley Soup*	Grant (2000)
Galen *De sanitate tuenda*	*Hygiene*	Johnston (2018)
Galen *De temperamentis*	*Mixtures*	Singer (1997)
Galen *Thrasybulus sive Utrum medicinae sit aut gymnasticae hygiene*	*Thrasybulus, whether Hygiene Belongs to Medicine or Physical Training*	Johnston (2018)

Author and title	English title	Edition and translation
Galen *De tranquillitate animi*	*Avoiding Distress*	Singer (2013)
Galen *De venae sectione adversus Erasistrateos Romae degentes*	*Bloodletting, against to Erasistrateans in Rome*	Brain (1986)
Hippocrates	*Aphorisms* *Regimen in Health* *Humours* *Regimen I, II, III* *Dreams*	Jones (1923), Volume 4
Hippocrates	*Prognostic* *Regimen in Acute Diseases*	Jones (1923), Volume 2
Hippocrates	*Epidemics I and III* *The Oath* *Nutriment*	Jones (1923), Volume 1
Hyginus *De munitionbus castrorum*	*Fortifying a Roman Camp*	Campbell (2018)
Justinian *Digesta*	*The Digest*	Scott (1932)
Livy *Ab urbe condita*	*History of Rome*	Foster (1989)
Lucian *Hippias*	*The Bath*	Harmon (1913)
Marcellus Empiricus *De medicamentis*	*On Medicines*	Helmreich (1889)
Marcus Aurelius	*Meditations*	Staniforth (1964)
Pausanias	*Description of Greece*	Jones (1918)
Pliny *Epistulae*	*Letters*	Radice (1963)
Pliny *Naturalis historia*	*Natural History*	Jones (1956)

Author and title	English title	Edition and translation
Plutarch *Quaestiones convivales*	*Table-Talk*	Clement and Hoffleit (1969)
Rufus of Ephesus *Quaestiones medicinales*	*Medical Questions*	Letts (2014)
Scribonius Largus *Compositiones medicamentorum*	*The Composition of Remedies*	Bernhold (1786) [in Latin]
Seneca *De beneficiis*	*On Benefits*	Basore (1928/1935)
Seneca *Epistulae morales ad Lucilium*	*Letters from a Stoic*	Campbell (2004)
Seneca *De ira*	*On Anger*	Basore (1928/1935)
Soranus *Gynaecia*	*Gynaecology*	Temkin (1956)
Strabo *Geographica*	*Geography*	Jones (1917/1932)
Suetonius *De vita Caesarum*	*The Twelve Caesars*	Graves (1957)
Tacitus *De vita Iulii Agricolae*	*The Agricola*	Mattingly and Handford (1970)
Tacitus *Annales*	*The Annals of Imperial Rome*	Grant (1973)
Tacitus *Historiae*	*The Histories*	Wellesley (1972)
Varro *De re rustica*	*On Agriculture*	Hooper and Ash (1935)
Vitruvius *De architectura*	*On Architecture*	Granger (1998)

Notes

Chapter 1
1. Summerton (2007).
2. Wright (1964).
3. Cunliffe (2000).
4. Carr (1961) pp. 3–26; Tosh (2010) pp. 118–174.
5. Tosh (2010) p. 33.

Chapter 2
1. Galen *De sanitate tuenda* 1: 1.
2. Galen *De sanitate tuenda*.
3. Johnson (2018) pp. xi–xx; Hippocrates *Regimen in Health*.
4. Arikha (2008) pp. 3–41; Hankinson (2008b).
5. Hippocrates *Regimen in Health*.
6. Arikha (2008) pp. 3–41; Hankinson (2008b).
7. Galen *De sanitate tuenda* 1: 5.
8. Emch-Dériaz (1992).
9. Galen *De sanitate tuenda* 1: 5.
10. Galen *De sanitate tuenda* 1: 5.
11. Galen *De sanitate tuenda* 1: 5.
12. Galen *Thrasybulus sive Utrum medicinae sit aut gymnasticae hygiene.*
13. Jarcho (1970).
14. Seneca *Epistulae morales ad Lucilium* 5.
15. Galen *Ars medica* 23.
16. Galen *De sanitate tuenda* 1: 15.
17. Galen *De sanitate tuenda* 5: 11.
18. Galen *De sanitate tuenda* 2: 1.

19. Galen *De sanitate tuenda* 1: 11.
20. Celsus *De medicina* 1: 2; 3.
21. Pliny *Epistulae* 5: 6.
22. Pliny *Epistulae* 2: 17.
23. Gilgen *et al.* (2019).
24. Seneca *Epistulae morales ad Lucilium* 104: 6.
25. Nutton (2020) p. 61; Debru (2008).
26. Galen *De sanitate tuenda* 1: 8.
27. Debru (2008).
28. Baker (2018).
29. Galen *De sanitate tuenda* 2: 2.
30. Galen *De sanitate tuenda* 2: 2.
31. Celsus *De medicina* 1: 2; 6.
32. Galen *De sanitate tuenda* 2: 11.
33. Galen *De sanitate tuenda* 2: 2.
34. Galen *De sanitate tuenda* 6: 14.
35. Vitruvius *De architectura* 5: 9; 5.
36. Galen *De sanitate tuenda* 5: 11.
37. Galen *De sanitate tuenda* 5: 1.
38. Galen *De sanitate tuenda* 2: 2; Celsus *De medicina* 1: 2; 7.
39. Celsus *De medicina* 1: 2; 6.
40. Galen *De sanitate tuenda* 5: 2.
41. Galen *De sanitate tuenda* 5: 3.
42. Celsus *De medicina* 1: 2; 7.
43. Galen *Thrasybulus sive Utrum medicinae sit aut gymnasticae hygiene* 41.
44. Galen *De parvae pilae exercitio.*
45. Galen *De sanitate tuenda* 2: 11.
46. Galen *De causis symptomatum* 1: 8.
47. Draycott (2019); Jashemski (1999).
48. Seneca *De ira* 3: 36.
49. Marcus Aurelius *Meditations* 5: 1.
50. Celsus *De medicina* 1: 2; 8.

51. Celsus *De medicina* 2: 18; 1.
52. http: //blogs.exeter.ac.uk/ancienthealthcare/.
53. Celsus *De medicina* 2: 18; 2–3; Jackson (1988) p. 34.
54. Galen *De causis morborum* 2: 2.
55. Hippocrates *Regimen in Health.*
56. Hippocrates *Regimen in Health.*
57. Galen *De sanitate tuenda* 1: 7.
58. Galen *De sanitate tuenda* 5: 4.
59. Grant (2000).
60. Bisel and Bisel (2002); Rowan (2014).
61. Rowan (2014).
62. Plutarch *Quaestiones convivales* 7: 9.
63. Seneca *Epistulae morales ad Lucilium* 108.
64. Grainger (2006).
65. Galen *De sanitate tuenda* 1: 6.
66. Hippocrates *Regimen in Health.*
67. Pliny *Naturalis historia* 23: 23.
68. Galen *De sanitate tuenda* 5: 2.
69. Galen *De alimentorum facultatibus* 2: 27.
70. Galen *De ptisana.*
71. Galen *De sanitate tuenda* 1: 12.
72. Curth (2003).
73. Galen *De sanitate tuenda* 2: 2; Celsus *De medicina* 1: 2; 4.
74. Cheyne (1724).
75. Galen *De sanitate tuenda.*
76. McLynn (2010) pp. 466–467; Littman and Littman (1973); Duncan-Jones (2018).
77. Galen *De libris propriis* 3: 3.
78. Summerton (2018).
79. Wargocki (2013).
80. Rowan (2014).
81. GBD 2017 Diet Collaborators (2019); Barnard (2019).
82. Tong *et al.* (2016).

83. Galen *De sanitate tuenda* 1: 5.
84. Galen *De constitutione artis medicae* 18.
85. Summerton (1999).
86. Summerton (2011).
87. Celsus *De medicina* 1: 3; 13.
88. Galen *De sanitate tuenda* 1: 5.
89. Rose (1992).
90. Stensvold *et al.* (2020).
91. Galen *De sanitate tuenda* 1: 5.
92. Celsus *De medicina* 1: 1; 1.
93. Emch-Dériaz (1992).
94. Korhonen *et al.* (2020).
95. Summerton (2018).
96. Galen *De sanitate tuenda* 5: 1.
97. Marsden *et al.* (2014).
98. http: //blogs.exeter.ac.uk/ancienthealthcare/.
99. Ilardi (2010).
100. http: //tlc.ku.edu/sites/tlc.drupal.ku.edu/files/files/PosterAPS2012.pdf.
101. Beeson (2019); Farrar (2011).
102. Pliny *Naturalis historia*.
103. Jashemski (1999).
104. Pliny *Naturalis historia* 25: 5.
105. Galen *De sanitate tuenda* 2: 8.
106. Pliny *Epistulae* 5: 6.
107. Price (2000).
108. Vitruvius *De architectura* 5: 9; 8.
109. Beeson (2019); Farrar (2011).
110. Farrar (2011) p. 53.
111. Pliny *Epistulae* 2: 17.
112. Galen *Ars medica* 23.
113. Soga *et al.* (2017).
114. Tester-Jones *et al.* (2020).

Chapter 3

1. Tomlin (1991); Bowman and Thomas (2003), letter 586, pp. 38–39.
2. Pliny *Epistulae* 10: 5.
3. Varo *De re rustica* 2:1; 21.
4. Bowman and Thomas (1994), letter 294, p. 264.
5. Israelowich (2015) pp. 11–19; Nutton (2013) pp. 160–164; Livy *Ab urbe condita* 10: 47.
6. Pliny *Naturalis historia* 29: 7.
7. Nutton (2013) pp. 166–167.
8. Israelowich (2015) pp. 21–22.
9. Tacitus *Annales* 12: 66.
10. Cooley and Cooley (2014) p. 110.
11. Montgomery *et al.* (2011).
12. Barnes (1914); Nutton (1968).
13. Scarth (1880).
14. Rémy (1984); Parker (1997).
15. Israelowich (2015) p. 17.
16. Rémy (1984).
17. Jackson (1988) p. 58; Nutton (2013) p. 196.
18. Ulpian in Justinian *Digesta* 50: 13; 1.
19. Scarborough (1969) pp. 122–133.
20. Nutton (2020) pp. 7–30; Galen *Quod optimus medicus sit quoque philosophus*.
21. Rémy (1984).
22. Rémy (1984).
23. Jackson (1988) pp. 58–59; Nutton (2013) pp. 254–278.
24. Rémy (1984).
25. Green (1955).
26. Nutton (2013) pp. 149–153.
27. Celsus *De medicina* Pro 36.
28. Hankinson (2008c); Nutton (2013) pp. 125–127.
29. Nutton (2013) pp. 191–206.

30. Rémy (1984).
31. Scarborough (1969) pp. 66–75.
32. Israelowich (2015) pp. 87–109; Nutton (1969).
33. Jackson (1988) pp. 126–137.
34. Allason-Jones (1999).
35. Barnes (1914); Gilson (1978).
36. Fox (1940).
37. Rémy (1984).
38. Israelowich (2015) pp. 105–106.
39. Bowman and Thomas (1994), letter 156, p. 100.
40. Celsus *De medicina* 6: 6; 1.
41. Pliny *Naturalis historia* 11: 52–54.
42. Birley (1992).
43. Baker (2011).
44. White and Barker (1998).
45. Baker (2011); Fauduet (1990).
46. Rothenhöfer (2018).
47. Boon (1983); Voinot (1999).
48. Jackson (1996).
49. Boon (1983); Voinot (1999); Baker (2011).
50. Boon (1983); Voinot (1999); Jackson (1996).
51. Jenkins (1986).
52. Hippocrates *Epidemics* 1: 23.
53. Nutton (2020) pp. 52–75.
54. Galen *De locus affectis* 5: 8.
55. Galen *De locus affectis* 5: 8.
56. Galen *De praecognitione* 7: 3.
57. Galen *De praecognitione* 6: 2.
58. Letts (2014).
59. Rufus of Ephesus *Quaestiones medicinales* 1 and 2: 1.
60. Letts (2014).
61. Celsus *De medicina* 3: 6; 6.
62. Morison (2008).

63. Morison (2008) p. 140.
64. Galen *De praecognitione* 6: 15.
65. Hart (1970).
66. Vauthey and Vauthey (1983).
67. Penn (1994) pp. 96–97.
68. Summerton (2011).
69. Rufus of Ephesus *Quaestiones medicinales* 15: 17.
70. Rufus of Ephesus *Quaestiones medicinales* 15: 15.
71. Morison (2008).
72. Seneca *De beneficiis* 6: 16; 2.
73. Hippocrates *Prognostics* 1.
74. Galen *De constitutione artis medicae* 17.
75. Galen *De constitutione artis medicae* 17.
76. Christakis (1999).
77. Schoenborn *et al.* (2016); Khuller and Jena (2016).
78. Hippocrates *Aphorisms* 2: 33.
79. St John and Montgomery (2014).
80. Thomas *et al.* (2019).
81. Galen *De constitutione artis medicae* 20.
82. Pliny *Naturalis historia* 29: 8; 17–18.
83. Nutton (2020) pp. 98–101; Scarborough (1969) pp. 114–115.
84. Soranus *Gynaecology* 1: 3.
85. Scribonius Largus *Compositiones medicamentorum* (*Epistula dedicatoria*).
86. Nutton (2020) pp. 98–131.
87. Galen *De praecognitione* 3: 3.
88. Israelowich (2015) pp. 28–29.
89. Justinian *Digesta* 50: 9; 1.
90. Israelowich (2015) pp. 30–32.
91. Askitopoulou and Vgontzas (2018a and 2018b); Antoniou *et al.* (2010); Oxtoby (2016).
92. Lucian *Hippias* 1.
93. Summerton (2000).

94. O'Neill (2002).
95. Pellegrino and Pellegrino (1988); Pellegrino (2006).

Chapter 4

1.   Roberts and Cox (2003) p. 124.
2.   McLynn (2010) pp. 466–467; Littman and Littman (1973); Duncan-Jones (2018).
3.   Dio Cassius *Historia Romana (Epitome)* 73: 14.
4.   Jones (2016).
5.   Hodgson and Breeze (2020).
6.   Simmonds *et al.* (2008).
7.   Millett (1990) pp. 185–186.
8.   Pliny *Epistulae* 10: 37.
9.   Tacitus *De vita Iulii Agricolae* 21.
10. Frontinus *De aquis urbis Romae* 1: 4.
11. Hodge (2002) p. 1.
12. Hodge (2002) pp. 161–170.
13. Hodge (2002) pp. 147–160.
14. Keenan-Jones *et al.* (2015).
15. De la Bédoyère (2001) pp. 213–214; Stephens (1985a); Stephens (1985b); Millett (1990) p. 106.
16. Jones (2002) pp. 96–98; Jones (2003), Wacher (1995) pp. 138–142.
17. Stephens (1985a).
18. Putnam (1997).
19. Williams (2003).
20. Jones (2003).
21. Mason (2001) p. 170.
22. Ottaway (2004) p. 43.
23. Crow (2004) pp. 41–45.
24. Charlier *et al.* (2012).
25. Hobson (2009) pp. 117–131.
26. Frontinus *De aquis urbis Romae* 2: 111.

27. White and Baker (1998).
28. Crow (2004) pp. 41–45.
29. Yegül (2010) pp. 101–132; Fagan (1999) pp. 104–118.
30. Yegül (2010) p. 3.
31. Aelius Aristides *Orationes* 15: 232.
32. Yegül (2010) pp. 101–132.
33. Fagan (1999) p. 272.
34. Fagan (1999) pp. 90–93.
35. Whitmore (2013).
36. Celsus *De medicina* 6: 6: 16.
37. Whitmore (2013); Voinot (1999).
38. Pliny *Epistulae* 9: 36.
39. Galen *De parvae pilae exertion.*
40. Yegül (2010) p. 246.
41. Seneca *Epistulae morales ad Lucilium* 56.
42. Yegül (2010); Fagan (1999); Rotherham (2012).
43. Jackson (1990a); Hodge (2002) p. 263; Soutelo (2014).
44. Tacitus *Historiae* 1: 67.
45. Celsus *De medicina* 2: 17.
46. Popkin (2018).
47. Soutelo (2014).
48. Jackson (1990a).
49. Voinot (1999).
50. Cunliffe (2000).
51. Jackson (1990a).
52. Pérez (2018).
53. Dunbabin (1989).
54. Seneca *Epistulae morales ad Lucilium* 86.
55. Fronto *Epistulae ad Marcum Caesarem* 1: 3.
56. Marcus Aurelius *Meditations* 8: 24.
57. Pliny *Naturalis historia* 11: 39.
58. Celsus *De medicina* 5: 26, 28.
59. Scobie (1986).

60. http: //jfbradu.free.fr/celtes/sceaux/sceaux-11.php3.
61. Dunbabin (1989).
62. Harvey (2016) p. 256.
63. Baker (2004) pp. 83–114.
64. Hyginus *De munitionbus castrorum* 4: 1.
65. Majno (1975) p. 387.
66. Crow (2004) pp. 54–55.
67. Cilliers and Retief (2002).
68. Cunliffe (2000).
69. Tacitus *Annales* 4: 63.
70. Downie *et al.* (1996).
71. Toynbee (1971) pp. 73–100.
72. Morley (2005) p. 198.
73. Ghebrehewet *et al.* (2016).
74. Frontinus *De aquis urbis Romae* Pref: 1.
75. Stephens (1985b).
76. Stephens (1985b).
77. Jones (2003).
78. Putnam (1997).
79. Mason (2001) p. 170; Ottaway (2004) p. 43; Jones (2002) pp. 56–57.
80. Stephens (1985a).
81. Scobie (1986).
82. Strabo *Geographica* 14: 1, 37.
83. Mitchell (2017).
84. Dobney (1999).
85. Scott *et al.* (2020).
86. Montgomery *et al.* (2010).
87. Majno (1975) p. 369.
88. Eisinger (1982).
89. Vitruvius *De architectura* 8: 6, 10.
90. Scobie (1986).
91. Braudel (1992) p. 310.

92. Millett (1990) p. 108.
93. Frontinus *De aquis urbis Romae* 1: 16.
94. https: //www.who.int/news-room/fact-sheets/detail/drinking-water.
95. https: //www.who.int/en/news-room/fact-sheets/detail/sanitation.
96. https: //unstats.un.org/sdgs/report/2019/goal-11/.
97. Vitruvius *De architectura* 1: 4, 1.
98. Vitruvius *De architectura* 1: 4, 9.
99. Vitruvius *De architectura* 5: 9, 5.
100. Pliny Epistulae 2: 17; Pliny Epistulae 5: 6; Columella De re rustica 1: 4, 9; Barefoot (2005).
101. Fagan (1999) p. 10.
102. Lucian *Hippias* 5: 7.
103. Golden *et al.* (2005).
104. Ulrich (2006).
105. Celsus *De medicina* Pro 65.
106. Edmond *et al.* (2017).
107. Ulrich (1984).
108. Ulrich (2006).
109. Hyginus *De munitionbus castrorum* 4: 1.
110. Ulrich (2006).

Chapter 5

1. Mann (1984) pp. 1–30.
2. Mann (1984) pp. 92–97; Petrovska (2012).
3. Galen *De temperamentis* 3: 2.
4. Totelin (2015).
5. Scribonius Largus *Compositiones medicamentorum* (*Epistula dedicatoria*).
6. Nutton (2013) pp. 175–178.
7. Mann (1984) p. 50.
8. Dioscorides *De materia medica*; Prioreschi (1998) pp. 236–244; Scarborough (1996); Nutton (2013) pp. 178–179.

9. Pliny *Naturalis historia*; Prioreschi (1998) pp. 220–229; van Tellingen (2007).
10. Pliny *Naturalis historia* 25: 6.
11. Fitzpatrick (1991).
12. Prioreschi (1998) p. 211.
13. Celsus *De medicina*.
14. Prioreschi (1998) p. 222.
15. Prioreschi (1998) pp. 433–435.
16. Nutton (2020) pp. 112–117.
17. Touwaide (2014).
18. Prioreschi (1998) pp. 433–435; Vogt (2008).
19. Jashemski (1999); Majno (1975) pp. 387–388.
20. Jackson (1988) p. 81.
21. Boon (1957) p. 99; Celsus *De medicina* 5: 5.
22. Jackson (1988) p. 82.
23. Boon (1957) p. 198.
24. Stacey (2011).
25. Jackson (1996); Boon (1983).
26. Jackson (1990b).
27. Freer and Tomlin (1992) pp. 48 and 52.
28. Voinot (1999).
29. Nielsen (1974) p. 62.
30. Boyer (1990).
31. Scribonius Largus *Compositiones medicamentorum* 33.
32. Marcellus Empiricus *De medicamentis* 8: 123 and 125.
33. Celsus *De medicina* 6: 6; 13.
34. Giachi *et al.* (2013).
35. Camden (1610).
36. Moog and Karenberg (2003).
37. Waller (1971).
38. Dioscorides *De materia medica* 1: 136.
39. Celsus *De medicina* 6: 18; 10.
40. Pliny *Naturalis historia* 24: 57.

41. Cato *De agri cultura* 157: 3.
42. Boi *et al.* (2012).
43. Boyer (1990).
44. Celsus *De medicina* 4: 28; 29.
45. https: //data.epo.org/gpi/EP1917018B1-Inulin-sulphate-for-the-treatment-of-osteoarthritis.
46. Bartels *et al.* (2006).
47. Harrison *et al.* (2012).
48. Littman and Littman (1973).
49. Dioscorides *De materia medica* 2: 101.
50. Celsus *De medicina* 5: 26; 29.
51. Mandal and Mandal (2011).
52. Eteraf-Oskouei and Najafi (2013).
53. Nielsen (1974).
54. Celsus *De medicina* 6: 6; 3.
55. Summerton (2013); Summerton (2015).
56. Harrison *et al.* (2015).
57. Furner-Pardoe *et al.* (2020).
58. http: //www.myrine.at/Gi/Gi_e.html.
59. Photos-Jones and Hall (2014).
60. Photos-Jones and Hall (2014); Photos-Jones (2018).
61. Liu and Liu (2016); Ji *et al.* (2009).
62. Connelly *et al.* (2020).
63. Prioreschi (1998) pp. 719–740.
64. Mann (1984) p. 95.
65. Harrison *et al.* (2015).
66. Boyer (1990).
67. Celsus *De medicina* 6: 6; 1.
68. Furner-Pardoe *et al.* (2020).
69. Pliny *Naturalis historia* 19: 125.
70. Dioscorides *De materia medica* 2: 136.
71. Celsus *De medicina* 2: 32.
72. Galen *De locis affectis* 2: 5.

73. Kim *et al.* (2017).
74. Celsus *De medicina* Pro 9.
75. Scribonius Largus *Compositiones medicamentorum* (*Epistula dedicatoria*).
76. https: //www.gov.uk/government/publications/prescribed-medicines-review-report/prescribed-medicines-review-summary.
77. Mann (1984) p. 50.
78. Nutton (2020) pp. 112–117.
79. https: //www.who.int/bulletin/volumes/88/4/10-020410/en/.
80. Scribonius Largus *Compositiones medicamentorum* (*Epistula dedicatoria*).
81. Galen *De methodo medendi* 14: 7.
82. Photos-Jones and Hall (2014).
83. Echt *et al.* (1991).
84. Furberg (2002).
85. Sackett *et al.* (1996).

Chapter 6

1. Galen *De praecognitione* 7: 3.
2. Irvine (2009); Robertson (2019).
3. Israelowich (2015) pp. 111–117.
4. Galen *De sanitate tuenda* 1: 8.
5. Hutchinson and Brawer (2011).
6. Israelowich (2015) p. 53.
7. Oberhelman (1983).
8. Downie (2013); Horstmanshoff (2004); Stephens (2012).
9. Singer (2013).
10. Galen *De tranquillitate animi* 54.
11. Galen *De tranquillitate animi* 48.
12. Irvine (2009) pp. 29–61.
13. Irvine (2009) pp. 44–61; Robertson (2019).
14. Epictetus *Encheiridion* 1.
15. Epictetus *Encheiridion* 5.

16. Marcus Aurelius *Meditations* 12: 22.
17. Marcus Aurelius *Meditations* 10: 34.
18. Marcus Aurelius *Meditations* 2: 1.
19. Hart (2000) pp. 1–51.
20. Hart (2000) pp. 53–77; Dio Cassius *Epitome* 78: 15; 6–7; van der Ploeg (2016).
21. Edelstein and Edelstein (1998); Hart (2000); Bertaux (1991); Wheeler and Wheeler (1932); Wightman (1970); Cunliffe (2000).
22. Hart (2000) pp. 79–90; Israelowich (2015) pp. 111–117.
23. Edelstein and Edelstein (1998) pp. 139–180.
24. Aelius Aristides *Orationes* 48: 34–35.
25. Hart (2000) pp. 41–51 and 59.
26. Charitonidou (1978).
27. Strabo *Geographica* 14: 1, 44.
28. Bertaux (1991).
29. Israelowich (2015) p. 53.
30. Pausanias *Description of Greece* 2: 27.
31. Casey *et al.* (1999); Wheeler and Wheeler (1932).
32. Wright (1985).
33. Edelstein and Edelstein (1998) p. 233.
34. Edelstein and Edelstein (1998) p. 234.
35. Edelstein and Edelstein (1998); Wheeler and Wheeler (1932); Hart (2000); Cilliers and Retief (2013).
36. Voinot (1999).
37. Cunliffe (2000).
38. Hart (1970).
39. Aelius Aristides *Orationes* 39: 14–15.
40. Edelstein and Edelstein (1998) pp. 208–213; Hartigan (2005).
41. Pausanias *Description of Greece* 1: 21; 4.
42. Edelstein and Edelstein (1998) p. 339; Wheeler and Wheeler (1932).
43. Edelstein and Edelstein (1998) pp. 199–208.
44. Green (1955).

45. Edelstein and Edelstein (1998) pp. 199–208.
46. Oberhelman (2014).
47. Oberhelman (1983).
48. Galen *Ars medica* 21.
49. Marcus Aurelius *Meditations* 2: 1.
50. Robertson (2019).
51. Marcus Aurelius *Meditations*.
52. Robertson (2019) p. 108.
53. Shakespeare (2007 ed.) Act 2, Scene 2.
54. Singer (2013); Seneca *Epistulae morales ad Lucilium*; Marcus Aurelius *Meditations*; Epictetus *Encheiridion*.
55. Irvine (2009) pp. 65–84 and 119–124.
56. Robertson (2010).
57. Epictetus *Encheiridion*.
58. Robertson (2010).
59. Edelstein and Edelstein (1998); Penn (1994).
60. Casey *et al.* (1999).
61. Dodds (1965).
62. Edelstein and Edelstein (1998).
63. Edelstein and Edelstein (1998) p. 364.
64. Nutton (2020) p. 87.
65. Angeletti *et al.* (1992).
66. Vitruvius *De architectura* 1: 2; 7.
67. Ammianus Marcellinus *Res Gestae* 22: 16; 14.
68. Barefoot (2005); Baker (2017).
69. Li (2019).
70. Aelius Aristides *Orationes* 47: 65.
71. Edelstein and Edelstein (1998) p. 248.
72. Cunliffe (2000).
73. Edelstein and Edelstein (1998) p. 248.
74. Aelius Aristides *Hieroi Logoi* 4: 2.
75. Edelstein and Edelstein (1998).
76. Dio Cassius *Epitome* 78: 15; 6–7.

77. Wightman (1970).
78. Walters (2009).
79. Bryn Walters (personal communication).
80. Don Macer-Wright (personal communication).
81. Charitonidou (1978).
82. Okay (2016).
83. Edelstein and Edelstein (1998); Hart (2000); Charitonidou (1978).
84. Cilliers and Retief (2013).
85. Okay (2016).
86. Edelstein and Edelstein (1998) pp. 163–164.
87. Edelstein and Edelstein (1998) p. 164.
88. Sturm *et al.* (2020).
89. Panagiotidou (2016).
90. Edelstein and Edelstein (1998) p. 202.
91. Hartigan (2005); Fancourt and Finn (2019).
92. Katz and Shapiro (1993).
93. Tick (2001); Dubisch (2013).
94. Cohen *et al.* (2017).

Chapter 7

1. Celsus *De medicina.*
2. Green (1955).
3. Jackson (2011) p. 249.
4. Milne (1907).
5. Celsus *De medicina* 7: 5; 3.
6. Majno (1975) p. 361.
7. Ratcliffe (2013).
8. Jackson (1995).
9. Taylor (2007).
10. Celsus *De medicina* 5: 26; 23A–B.
11. Majno (1975) pp. 365–367; Ratcliffe (2013).
12. Celsus *De medicina* 5: 26; 23D.

13. Ratcliffe (2013).
14. Celsus *De medicina* 7: 31; 1.
15. Ratcliffe (2013).
16. Celsus *De medicina* 7: 12; 2.
17. Adoga and Nimkur (2011).
18. Celsus *De medicina* 7: 12; 2; Thomas (1963).
19. Boon (1991).
20. Jackson (1997); Baker (2004) p. 5.
21. White and Barker (1998).
22. Celsus *De medicina* 8: 10; 7F–G.
23. Thomas (1963).
24. Celsus *De medicina* Pro 30.
25. Jackson (2011) p. 251.
26. Jackson (2014).
27. Jackson and La Niece (1986).
28. Ratcliffe (2013).
29. Jackson, personal communication.
30. Jackson and Leahy (1990).
31. Boon (1957).
32. Celsus *De medicina* 8: 3; 1.
33. Celsus *De medicina* 8: 3; 2–3.
34. Jackson (2005) p. 108.
35. Tullo (2010).
36. Taylor (2007).
37. Jackson (2002).
38. Jackson (2003).
39. Celsus *De medicina* 7: 7; 14.
40. Jackson (1990c); Jackson (2011) p. 257.
41. Fagan (1999).
42. Celsus *De medicina* 2: 17.
43. Celsus *De medicina* 2: 17.
44. Celsus *De medicina* 2: 17.
45. Green (1955).

46. Suetonius *De vita Caesarum* Augustus: 81.
47. Green (1955).
48. Pliny *Naturalis historia* 31: 2.
49. Vitruvius *De architectura* 8: 3; 4.
50. Jackson (1990a).
51. Galen *De sanitate tuenda* 2: 4.
52. Galen *De sanitate tuenda* 2: 3.
53. Celsus *De medicina* 2: 14; 2.
54. Celsus *De medicina* 2: 14; 8.
55. Celsus *De medicina* 2: 15; 1.
56. Celsus *De medicina* 2: 15; 3.
57. Brain (1986).
58. Celsus *De medicina* 2: 11; 3.
59. Brain (1986); Papavramidou and Christopoulou-Aletra (2009).
60. Galen *De venae sectione adversus Erasistrateos Romae degentes* 60.
61. Meade *et al.* (1990).
62. Scarborough (1969) p. 86.
63. Galen *De tranquillitate animi* 4–5.
64. Jackson and La Niece (1986).
65. Wells (1967).
66. Celsus *De medicina* 2: 11; 3; Ratcliffe (2013).
67. Boyer (1990).
68. http: //videotheque.cnrs.fr/doc=607.
69. Royal College of Surgeons, Professional Standards (2019).
70. Scarborough (1969) p. 99.
71. Rocca (2008) p. 242.
72. Ratcliffe (2013).
73. Nutton (2020) p. 112.
74. Celsus *De medicina* 7: 12; 2.
75. Celsus *De medicina* 3: 10; 2.
76. Galen *De method medendi* 6: 6.
77. Stewart *et al.* (2012); Kamal *et al.* (2017).

78. Volpp *et al.* (2012).
79. Mooventhan and Nivethitha (2014).
80. Bartels *et al.* (2016).
81. Kohara *et al.* (2018); Laukkanen *et al.* (2018).
82. Lebert (2020).
83. Cherkin *et al.* (2011).
84. Perlman *et al.* (2012).
85. Watson *et al.* (1998); Cross *et al.* (2018).
86. Kim *et al.* (2011).
87. Greenstone (2010); Houschyar *et al.* (2012).

Chapter 8
1. Green (1955) p. 47.
2. Reilly *et al.* (2018).

Bibliography

Adoga AA and Nimkur TL (2011). The traditionally amputated uvula amongst Nigerians: Still an ongoing practice. *ISRN Otolaryngology*: 704924. https://doi.org/10.5402/2011/704924

Allason-Jones L (1999). Health Care in the Roman North. *Britannia* 30: pp. 133–146.

Angeletti L, Agrimi U, French D, *et al*. (1992). Healing rituals and sacred serpents. *Lancet* 340: pp. 223–225.

Antoniou SA, Antoniou GA, Granderath FA, *et al*. (2010). Reflections of the Hippocratic Oath in modern medicine. *World Journal of Surgery* 34: pp. 3075–3079.

Arikha N (2008). *Passions and Tempers. A History of the Humours*. New York: Harper Perennial.

Ash HB (1941). *Columella: On Agriculture (Loeb Classical Library)*. Cambridge, MA: Harvard University Press.

Askitopoulou H and Vgontzas AN (2018a). The relevance of the Hippocratic Oath to the ethical and moral values of contemporary medicine. Part I: The Hippocratic Oath from antiquity to modern times. *European Spine Journal* 27: pp. 1481–1490.

Askitopoulou H and Vgontzas AN (2018b). The relevance of the Hippocratic Oath to the ethical and moral values of contemporary medicine. Part II: interpretation of the Hippocratic Oath – today's perspective. *European Spine Journal* 27: pp. 1491–1500.

Baker PA (2004). *Medical Care for the Roman Army on the Rhine, Danube and British Frontiers in the First, Second and Early Third Centuries AD. BAR International Series 1286*. Oxford: Hadrian Books.

Baker PA (2011). Collyrium stamps: An indicator of regional practices in Roman Gaul. *European Journal of Archaeology* 14: pp. 158–189.

Baker PA (2017). Viewing health: Asclepia in their natural settings. *Religion in the Roman Empire* 3: pp. 143–163.

Baker PA (2018). Identifying the connection between Roman conceptions of 'Pure Air' and physical and mental health in Pompeian gardens (c.150 BC–AD 79): A multi-sensory approach to ancient medicine. *World Archaeology* 50: pp. 404–417.

Barefoot P (2005). Buildings for health: Then and now, in H King (ed.). *Health in Antiquity.* Abingdon: Routledge, pp. 205–215.

Barnard ND (2019). Ignorance of nutrition is no longer defensible. *JAMA Intern Med* 179: pp. 1021–1022.

Barnes H (1914). On Roman medicine and Roman medical inscriptions found in Britain. *Proc. R. Soc. Med.* 7: pp. 71–87.

Bartels EM, Swaddling J, Harrison AP (2006). An ancient Greek pain remedy for athletes. *Pain Practice* 6: pp. 212–218.

Bartels EM, Juhl CB, Christensen R, *et al.* (2016). Aquatic exercise for the treatment of knee and hip osteoarthritis. *Cochrane Database Syst Rev.* 3: CD005523.

Basore JW (1928/1935). *Seneca: Moral Essays (Loeb Classical Library).* Cambridge, MA: Harvard University Press.

Beck LY (2005). *De materia medica by Pedanius Dioscorides.* Hildesheim, Germany: Olms-Weidmann.

Beeson A (2019). *Roman Gardens.* Stroud: Amberley.

Behr CA (1981 and 1986). *P. Aelius Aristides: The Complete Works.* Leiden: Brill.

Bennett CE (1925). *Frontinus: Stratagems; Aqueducts of Rome (Loeb Classical Library).* Cambridge, MA: Harvard University Press.

Bernhold JM (1786). *Scribonii Largi. Compositiones Medicamentorum.* Milton Keynes: Lightening Source.

Bertaux C (1991). Grand. Prestigieux sanctuaire de la Gaule. Divinities et cultes antiques. *Les Dossiers d'Archeologie* 162: pp. 42–49.

Birley AR (1992). A case of eye disease (Lippitudo) on the Roman frontier in Britain. *Documenta Ophthalmologica* 81: pp. 111–119.

Bisel SC and Bisel JF (2002). Health and nutrition at Herculaneum: An examination of human skeletal remains, in W Jashemski and F Meyer (eds). *The Natural History of Pompeii*. Cambridge: Cambridge University Press, pp. 451–475.

Boi B, Koh S, Gail D (2012). The effectiveness of cabbage leaf application (treatment) on pain and hardness in breast engorgement and its effect on the duration of breastfeeding. *JBI Database of Systematic Reviews and Implementation Reports* 10: pp. 1185–1213.

Boon G (1957). *Roman Silchester*. London: Max Parrish.

Boon G (1983). Potters, oculists and eye-troubles. *Britannia* 14: pp. 1–12.

Boon G (1991). 'Tonsor humanus': Razor and toilet-knife in antiquity. *Britannia* 22: pp. 21–32.

Bowman AK and Thomas JD (1994). *The Vindolanda Writing Tablets (Tabulae Vindolandenses) – Volume 2*. London: British Museum Press.

Bowman AK and Thomas JD (2003). *The Vindolanda Writing Tablets (Tabulae Vindolandenses) – Volume 3*. London: British Museum Press.

Boyer R (1990). Découverte de la tombe d'un oculiste à Lyon. *Gallia* 47: pp. 215–249.

Brain P (1986). *Galen on Bloodletting*. Cambridge: Cambridge University Press.

Braudel F (1992). *The Structures of Everyday Life. Civilization and Capitalism 15th–18th Century*. London: Fontana.

Camden W (1610). *Britain, or, a Chorographicall Description of the Most Flourishing Kingdomes, England, Scotland, and Ireland*. London: George Bishop and John Norton.

Campbell DB (2018). *Fortifying a Roman Camp. The Liber de munitionibus castrorum of Hyginus*. Glasgow: Bocca della Verita.

Campbell R (2004). *Seneca: Letters from a Stoic*. London: Penguin.

Carr EH (1961). *What Is History?* London: Penguin.

Casey P, Hoffmann B, Dore J (1999). Excavations at the Roman Temple in Lydney Park, Gloucestershire in 1980 and 1981. *The Antiquaries Journal* 79: pp. 81–143.

Charitonidou A (1978). *Epidaurus*. Belgrade: Clio.

Charlier P, Brun L, Prêtre C, Huynh-Charlier I (2012). Toilet hygiene in the classical era. *British Medical Journal* 345: p. 41.

Cherkin DC, Sherman KJ, Kahn J, *et al.* (2011). A comparison of the effects of 2 types of massage and usual care on chronic low back pain: A randomized, controlled trial. *Annals of Internal Medicine* 155: pp. 1–9.

Cheyne G (1724). *An Essay of Health and Long Life.* London: George Strahan.

Christakis NA (1999). *Death Foretold. Prophecy and Prognosis in Medical Care.* Chicago: University of Chicago Press.

Cilliers L and Retief FP (2002). The evolution of the hospital from antiquity to the end of the middle ages. *Curationis* 25: pp. 60–66.

Cilliers L and Retief FP (2013). Dream healing in Asclepieia in the Mediterranean, in SM Oberhelman (ed.). *Dreams, Healing and Medicine in Greece.* Farnham: Ashgate, pp. 69–92.

Clement PA and Hoffleit HB (1969). *Plutarch. Moralia, Volume VIII: Table-Talk, Books 1–6 (Loeb Classical Library).* Cambridge, MA: Harvard University Press.

Cohen MM, Elliott F, Oates L, *et al.* (2017). Do wellness tourists get well? An observational study of multiple dimensions of health and well-being after a week-long retreat. *Journal of Alternative and Complementary Medicine* 23: pp. 140–148.

Connelly E, del Genio CI, Harrison F (2020). Data mining a medieval medical text reveals patterns in ingredient choice that reflect biological activity against infectious agents. *mBio* 11: e03136–19.

Cooley AE and Cooley MGL (2014). *Pompeii and Herculaneum: A Sourcebook.* London: Routledge.

Cross RL, White J, Engelsher J, O'Connor SS (2018). Implementation of rocking chair therapy for veterans in residential substance use disorder treatment. *Journal of the American Psychiatric Nurses Association* 24: pp. 190–198.

Crow J (2004). *Housesteads. A Fort and Garrison on Hadrian's Wall.* Stroud: Tempus.

Cruse A (2004). *Roman Medicine.* Stroud: Tempus.

Cunliffe B (2000). *Roman Bath Discovered.* Stroud: Tempus.

Curth L (2003). Lessons from the past: Preventive medicine in early modern England. *Medical Humanities* 29: pp. 16–20.

De la Bédoyère (2001). *The Buildings of Roman Britain.* Stroud: Tempus.

Debru A (2008). Physiology, in RJ Hankinson (ed.). *The Cambridge Companion to Galen.* Cambridge: Cambridge University Press, pp. 263–282.

Dobney K, Hall A and Kenward H (1999). It's all garbage … A review of bioarchaeology in the four English *colonia* towns, in HR Hirst (ed.). *The* Coloniae *of Roman Britain.* Journal of Roman Archaeology, Supplementary Series 36. Portsmouth: RI, pp. 15–35.

Dodds ER (1965). *Pagan and Christian in an Age of Anxiety.* Cambridge: Cambridge University Press.

Downie J (2013). Dream hermeneutics in Aelius Aristides' *Hieroi Logoi*, in SM Oberhelman (ed.). *Dreams, Healing and Medicine in Greece.* Farnham: Ashgate, pp. 109–127.

Downie RS, Tannahill C, Tannahill A (1996). *Health Promotion. Models and Values.* Oxford: Oxford University Press.

Draycott J (2019). *Roman Domestic Medical Practice in Central Italy: From the Middle Republic to the Early Empire.* Abingdon: Routledge.

Dubisch J (2013). Dream healing for a new age, in SM Oberhelman (ed.). *Dreams, Healing and Medicine in Greece.* Farnham: Ashgate, pp. 317–331.

Dunbabin KMD (1989). Baiarum grata voluptas: Pleasures and dangers of the baths. *Papers of the British School at Rome* 57: pp. 6–46.

Duncan-Jones RP (2018). The Antonine Plague revisited. *Arctos* 52: pp. 41–72.

Echt DS, Liebson PR, Mitchell LB, *et al.* (1991). Mortality and morbidity in patients receiving encainide, flecainide, or placebo. The Cardiac Arrhythmia Suppression Trial. *The New England Journal of Medicine* 324: pp. 781–788.

Edelstein EJ and Edelstein L (1998). *Asclepius. Collection and Interpretation of the Testimonies.* Baltimore: John Hopkins University Press.

Edmond CYU, Pryor GA, Parker MJ (2017). Hospital at home – a review of our experience. *SICOT J* 3: pp. 60–65.

Eisinger J (1982). Lead and wine: Eberhard Gockel and the Colica Pictonum. *Medical History* 26: pp. 279–302.

Emch-Dériaz A (1992). The non-naturals made easy, in R Porter (ed.). *The Popularization of Medicine 1650–1850.* Abingdon: Routledge. pp. 134–159.

Eteraf-Oskouei T and Najafi M (2013). Traditional and modern uses of natural honey in human diseases: A review. *Iranian Journal of Basic Medical Sciences* 16: pp. 731–742.

Fagan GG (1999). *Bathing in Public in the Roman World.* Ann Arbor: University of Michigan Press.

Fancourt D and Finn S (2019). *What Is the Evidence on the Role of the Arts in Improving Health and Well-being? A Scoping Review. Health Evidence Network (HEN) Synthesis Report.* Copenhagen: WHO Regional Office for Europe.

Farrar L (2011). *Ancient Roman Gardens.* Stroud: History Press.

Fauduet I (1990). Les ex-voto anatomiques du sanctuaire de Bû. *Revue Archéologique de l'Ouest* 7: pp. 93–100.

Fitzpatrick A (1991). Ex Radice Britanica. *Britannia* 22: pp. 143–146.

Foster BO (1989). *Livy: History of Rome (Loeb Classical Library).* Cambridge, MA: Harvard University Press.

Foster HB (1914). *Dio Cassius: Roman History (Loeb Classical Library).* Cambridge, MA: Harvard University Press.

Fox A (1940). The legionary fortress at Caerleon in Monmouthshire: Excavations at Myrtle Cottage Orchard 1939. *Archaeologia Cambriensis* 95: pp. 101–152.

Freer SS and Tomlin RSO (eds) (1992). *The Roman Inscriptions of Britain. Volume II. Instrumentum Domesticum.* Stroud: Alan Sutton.

Furberg CD (2002). To whom do the research findings apply? *Heart* 87: pp. 570–574.

Furner-Pardoe J, Anonye BO, Cain R. *et al.* (2020). Anti-biofilm efficacy of a medieval treatment for bacterial infection requires the combination of multiple ingredients. *Sci Rep* 10: 12687. https://doi.org/10.1038/s41598-020-69273-8.

GBD 2017 Diet Collaborators (2019). Health effects of dietary risks in 195 countries, 1990–2017: A systematic analysis for the Global Burden of Disease Study 2017. *Lancet* 393: pp. 1958–1972.

Ghebrehewet S, Stewart AG, Baxter D, *et al.* (2016). *Health Protection: Principles and Practice.* Oxford: Oxford University Press.

Giachi G, Pallecchi P, Romualdi A, *et al.* (2013). Ingredients of a 2,000-y-old medicine revealed by chemical, mineralogical, and botanical investigations. *Proceedings of the National Academy of Sciences* 110: pp. 1193–1196.

Gilgen A, Wilkenskjeld S, Kaplan JO, *et al.* (2019). Effects of land use and anthropogenic aerosol emissions in the Roman Empire. *Climate of the Past* 15, pp. 1885–1911.

Gilson A (1978). A doctor at housesteads. *Archaeologia Aeliana* 6: pp. 162–165.

Golden RN, Gaynes BN, Ekstrom RD, *et al.* (2005). The efficacy of light therapy in the treatment of mood disorders: A review and meta-analysis of the evidence. *Am J Psychiatry* 162: pp. 656–662.

Granger F (1998). *Vitruvius: On Architecture (Loeb Classical Library).* Cambridge, MA: Harvard University Press.

Grainger S (2006). *Cooking Apicius: Roman Recipes for Today.* Totnes: Prospect Books.

Grant M (1973). *Tacitus: The Annals of Imperial Rome*. London: Penguin.

Grant M (2000). *Galen on Food and Diet*. Abingdon: Routledge.

Graves R (1957). *Suetonius: The Twelve Caesars*. London: Penguin.

Green RM (1955). *Asclepiades. His Life and Writings*. New Haven: Licht.

Greenstone G (2010). The history of bloodletting. *British Columbia Medical Journal*. 52: pp. 12–14.

Haines CR (1919). *The Correspondence of Marcus Cornelius Fronto*. London: Heinemann.

Harmon AM (1913). *Lucian: Hippias or The Bath (Loeb Classical Library)*. Cambridge, MA: Harvard University Press.

Hankinson RJ (2008a). *The Cambridge Companion to Galen*. Cambridge: Cambridge University Press.

Hankinson RJ (2008b). Philosophy of Nature, in RJ Hankinson (ed.). *The Cambridge Companion to Galen*. Cambridge: Cambridge University Press, pp. 210–241.

Hankinson RJ (2008c). Epistemology, in RJ Hankinson (ed.). *The Cambridge Companion to Galen*. Cambridge: Cambridge University Press, pp. 157–183.

Harrison AP, Hansen SH, Bartels EM (2012). Transdermal opioid patches for pain treatment in Ancient Greece. *Pain Practice* 12: pp. 620–625.

Harrison F, Roberts AE, Gabrilska R, *et al*. (2015). A 1,000-year-old antimicrobial remedy with antistaphylococcal activity. *mBio* 6: e01129.

Hart G (1970). A hematological artifact from 4th century Britain. *Bulletin of the History of Medicine* 44: pp. 76–79.

Hart G (2000). *Asclepius the God of Medicine*. London: Royal Society of Medicine.

Hartigan K (2005). Drama and healing: Ancient and modern, in H King (ed.). *Health in Antiquity*. London: Routledge, pp. 162–179.

Harvey BK (2016). *Daily Life in Ancient Rome: A Sourcebook.* Indianapolis: Hackett.

Helmreich G (1889). *Marcelli: De medicamentis.* Leipzig: Teubner.

Hobson B (2009). *Latrinae et Foricae. Toilets in the Roman World.* London: Duckworth.

Hodge AT (2002). *Roman Aqueducts & Water Supply.* London: Duckworth.

Hodgson N and Breeze D (2020). Plague on Hadrian's Wall? Interpreting evidence for pandemics in Roman Britain. *Current Archaeology* 365: pp. 28–35.

Hooper WD and Ash HB (1935). *Cato and Varro on Agriculture (Loeb Classical Library).* Cambridge, MA: Harvard University Press.

Horstmanshoff HF (2004). Asclepius and temple medicine in Aelius Aristides' Sacred Tales. *Studies in Ancient Medicine* 27: pp. 325–341.

Houschyar KS, Lüdtke R, Dobos GJ, *et al.* (2012). Effects of phlebotomy-induced reduction of body iron stores on metabolic syndrome: Results from a randomized clinical trial. *BMC Med* 10: 54. https://doi.org/10.1186/1741-7015-10-54.

Hulskamp MA (2013). The value of dream diagnosis in the medical praxis of the Hippocratics and Galen, in SM Oberhelman (ed.). *Dreams, Healing and Medicine in Greece.* Farnham: Ashgate, pp. 33–68.

Hutchinson TA and Brawer JR (2011). The challenge of medical dichotomies and the congruent physician–patient relationship in medicine, in TA Hutchinson (ed.). *Whole Person Care. A New Paradigm for the 21st Century.* London: Springer, pp. 31–43.

Ilardi S (2010). *The Depression Cure: The Six-Step Programme to Beat Depression Without Drugs.* London: Ebury.

Irvine WB (2009). *A Guide to the Good Life. The Ancient Art of Stoic Joy.* Oxford: Oxford University Press.

Israelowich I (2015). *Patients and Healers in the High Roman Empire.* Baltimore: John Hopkins University Press.

Jackson R and La Niece S (1986). A set of Roman medical instruments from Italy. *Britannia* 17: pp. 119–167.

Jackson R (1988). *Doctors and Diseases in the Roman Empire*. London: British Museum Publications.

Jackson R (1990a). Waters and spas in the classical world. *Medical History, Supplement* 10: pp. 1–13.

Jackson R (1990b). A new collyrium stamp from Cambridge and a correct reading of the stamp from Caistor-by-Norwich. *Britannia* 21: pp. 275–283.

Jackson R (1990c). Roman doctors and their Instruments: Recent research into ancient practice. *Journal of Roman Archaeology* 3: pp. 5–27.

Jackson R and Leahy K (1990). A Roman surgical forceps from near Littleborough and a note on the type. *Britannia* 21: pp. 271–274.

Jackson R (1995). The composition of Roman medical instrumentaria as an indicator of medical practice: A provisional assessment in *Ancient Medicine in its Socio-Cultural Context Vol. I*, P. van der Eijk, H. Horstmanshoff and P Schrijvers (eds). Amsterdam, Rodopi, pp. 189–207.

Jackson R (1996). A new collyrium stamp from Staines and some thoughts on eye medicine in Roman London and Britannia, in Bird J, Hassall M and Sheldon H (eds). *Interpreting Roman London: Papers in Memory of Hugh Chapman*. Oxford: Oxbow Monograph 58, pp. 177–187.

Jackson R (1997). An ancient British medical kit from Stanway, Essex. *Lancet* 350: pp. 1471–1473.

Jackson R (2002). A Roman doctors' house in Rimini. *British Museum Magazine* 44 pp. 20–23.

Jackson R (2003). The Domus 'del chirurgo' at Rimini: An interim account of the medical assemblage. *Journal of Roman Archaeology* 16: pp. 312–321.

Jackson R (2005). Holding onto health? Bone surgery and instrumentation in the Roman Empire, in H King (ed.). *Health in Antiquity*. Abingdon: Routledge, pp. 97–119.

Jackson R (2011). Medicine and hygiene, in L Allason-Jones (ed.). *Artefacts in Roman Britain. Their Purpose and Use*. Cambridge: Cambridge University Press, pp. 243–268.

Jackson R (2014). Back to basics: Surgeons' knives in the Roman world, in D Michaelides (ed.). *Medicine and Healing in the Ancient Mediterranean World*. Oxford: Oxbow Books, pp. 130–144.

Jarcho S (1970). Galen's six non-naturals: A bibliographic note and translation. *Bulletin of the History of Medicine* 44: pp. 372–377.

Jashemski WF (1999). *A Pompeian Herbal*. Austin: University of Texas Press.

Jenkins I (1986). *Greek and Roman Life*. London: British Museum Press.

Ji HF, Li XJ, Zhang HY (2009). Natural products and drug discovery. Can thousands of years of ancient medical knowledge lead us to new and powerful drug combinations in the fight against cancer and dementia? *EMBO reports* 10: pp. 194–200.

Johnson I (2006). *Galen: On Diseases and Symptoms*. Cambridge: Cambridge University Press.

Johnson I and Horsley GHR (2011). *Galen: Method of Medicine (Loeb Classical Library)*. Cambridge, MA: Harvard University Press.

Johnson I (2016). *Galen: On the Constitution of the Art of Medicine; The Art of Medicine; A Method of Medicine to Glaucon (Loeb Classical Library)*. Cambridge, MA: Harvard University Press.

Johnson I (2018). *Galen: Hygiene; Thrasybulus; On Exercise with a Small Ball (Loeb Classical Library)*. Cambridge, MA: Harvard University Press.

Jones CP (2016). An amulet from London and events surrounding the Antonine Plague. *Journal of Roman Archaeology* 29: pp. 469–472.

Jones HL (1917/1932). *The Geography of Strabo: In Eight Volumes (Loeb Classical Library)*. Cambridge, MA: Harvard University Press.

Jones MJ (2002). *Roman Lincoln: Conquest, Colony & Capital*. Stroud: Tempus.

Jones MJ (2003). Sources of effluence: Water through Roman Lincoln, in P Wilson (ed.). *The Archaeology of Roman Towns: Studies in Honour of John S. Wacher.* Oxford: Oxbow Books, pp. 111–127.

Jones WHS (1918). *Pausanias: Description of Greece (Loeb Classical Library).* Cambridge, MA: Harvard University Press.

Jones WHS (1923). *Hippocrates: Volumes 1–8 (Loeb Classical Library).* Cambridge, MA: Harvard University Press.

Jones WHS (1956). *Pliny: Natural History; Volumes 1–10 (Loeb Classical Library).* Cambridge, MA: Harvard University Press.

Kamal A, Akhuemonkhan E, Akshintala V, *et al.* (2017). Effectiveness of guideline-recommended cholecystectomy to prevent recurrent pancreatitis. *American Journal of Gastroenterology* 112: pp. 503–510.

Katz M and Shapiro CM (1993). Dreams and medical illness. *British Medical Journal* 306: pp. 993–995.

Keenan-Jones D, Motta D, Garcia MH, Fouke BW (2015). Travertine-based estimates of the amount of water supplied by ancient Rome's Anio Novus aqueduct. *Journal of Archaeological Science Reports* 3: pp. 1–10.

Khullar D, Jena AB (2016). Reducing prognostic errors: A new imperative in quality healthcare. *British Medical Journal* 352: pp. 66–67.

Kim JI, Lee MS, Lee DH, *et al.* (2011). Cupping for treating pain: A systematic review. *Evidence-Based Complementary and Alternative Medicine eCAM:* 467014. https://doi.org/10.1093/ecam/nep035.

Kim HD, Hong KB, Noh DO, Suh HJ (2017). Sleep-inducing effect of lettuce (*Lactuca sativa*) varieties on pentobarbital-induced sleep. *Food Sci Biotechnol.* 26: pp. 807–814.

Kohara K, Tabara Y, Ochi M, *et al.* (2018). Habitual hot water bathing protects cardiovascular function in middle-aged to elderly Japanese subjects. *Scientific Reports* 8: 10.1038/s41598-018-26908-1.

Korhonen M, Pentti J, Hartikainen J, *et al.* (2020). Lifestyle changes in relation to initiation of antihypertensive and lipid-lowering medication: A cohort study. *Journal of the American Heart Association* 9: e014168. 10.1161/JAHA.119.014168.

Laukkanen JA, Laukkanen T, Kunutsor SK (2018). Cardiovascular and other health benefits of sauna bathing: A review of the evidence. *Mayo Clinic Proceedings* 93: pp. 1111–1121.

Lebert R (2020). *Evidence-Based Massage Therapy: A Guide for Clinical Practice.* https://ecampusontario.pressbooks.pub/handbookformassagetherapists/.

Letts M (2014). Rufus of Ephesus and the patient's perspective in medicine. *British Journal for the History of Philosophy* 22: pp. 996–1020.

Li Q (2019). *Into the Forest: How Trees Can Help You Find Health and Happiness.* London: Penguin.

Littman RJ and Littman ML (1973). Galen and the Antonine Plague. *The American Journal of Philology* 94: pp. 243–255.

Liu W and Liu Y (2016). Youyou Tu: significance of winning the 2015 Nobel Prize in physiology or medicine. *Cardiovascular Diagnosis and Therapy* 6: pp. 1–2.

Long AA (2018). *How to be Free. An Ancient Guide to the Stoic Life.* Princeton: Princeton University Press.

Majno G (1975). *The Healing Hand. Man and Wound in the Ancient World.* Cambridge: Harvard University Press.

Mandal MD and Mandal S (2011). Honey: Its medicinal property and antibacterial activity. *Asian Pacific Journal of Tropical Biomedicine* 1: pp. 154–160.

Mann RD (1984). *Modern Drug Use. An Enquiry on Historical Principles.* Lancaster: MTP Press.

Marsden D, Wilkins J, Gill C, Dieppe P (2014). Galen and wellbeing: Whole person care. *International Journal of Whole Person Care* 1: pp. 76–78.

Mason DJP (2001). *Roman Chester: City of Eagles.* Stroud: Tempus.

Mattingly H and Handford SA (1970). *Tacitus: The Agricola and the Germania.* London: Penguin.

Meade TW, Dyer S, Browne W, *et al.* (1990). Low back pain of mechanical origin: Randomised comparison of chiropractic and hospital outpatient treatment. *British Medical Journal* 300: pp. 1431–1437.

McLynn F (2010). *Marcus Aurelius. Warrior, Philosopher, Emperor.* London: Vintage.

Millett M (1990). *The Romanization of Britain.* Cambridge: Cambridge University Press.

Milne JS (1907). *Surgical Instruments in Greek and Roman Times.* Oxford: Clarendon Press.

Mitchell PD (2017). Human parasites in the Roman World: Health consequences of conquering an empire. *Parasitology* 144: pp. 48–58.

Montgomery J, Evans JA, Chenery SR, *et al.* (2010). Gleaming, white and deadly: Using lead to track human exposure and geographic origins in the Roman period in Britain. *Journal of Roman archaeology; supplementary series*, Suppl. 78: pp. 199–226.

Montgomery J, Knüsel C, Tucker K (2011). Identifying the origins of decapitated male skeletons from 3 Driffield Terrace, York, through isotope analysis: Reflections of the cosmopolitan nature of Roman York in the time of Caracalla, in *The Bioarchaeology of the Human Head: Decapitation, Decoration and Deformation.* Gainesville, FL: University Press of Florida, pp. 141–178.

Moog F and Karenberg A (2003). Between horror and hope: Gladiator's blood as a cure for epileptics in ancient medicine. *Journal of the History of the Neurosciences* 12: pp. 137–143.

Mooventhan A and Nivethitha L (2014). Scientific evidence-based effects of hydrotherapy on various systems of the body. *North American Journal of Medical Sciences* 6: pp. 199–209.

Morison B (2008). Language, in RJ Hankinson (ed.). *The Cambridge Companion to Galen.* Cambridge: Cambridge University Press, pp. 116–156.

Morley N (2005). The salubriousness of the Roman City, in H King (ed.). *Health in Antiquity.* Abingdon: Routledge, pp. 192–204.

Nielsen H (1974). *Ancient Ophthalmological Agents: A Pharmaco-Historical Study of the Collyria and Seals for Collyria Used during*

Roman Antiquity, as well as of the Most Frequent Components of the Collyria. Odense: Odense University Press.

Nutton V (1968). A Greek doctor in Chester. *J Chester Archaeol. Soc.* 55: pp. 7–13.

Nutton V (1969). Medicine and the Roman army: A further reconsideration. *Medical History* 13: pp. 260–270.

Nutton V (1979). *Galen: On Prognosis.* Berlin: Akademie-Verlag.

Nutton V (2013). *Ancient Medicine.* London: Routledge.

Nutton V (2020). *Galen. A Thinking Doctor in Imperial Rome.* London: Routledge.

O'Neill O (2002). *A Question of Trust. The BBC Reith Lectures 2002.* Cambridge: Cambridge University Press.

Oberhelman SM (1983). Galen, on diagnosis from dreams. *Journal of the History of Medicine* 38: pp. 36–47.

Oberhelman SM (2014). Anatomical votive reliefs as evidence for specialization at healing sanctuaries in the ancient Mediterranean world. *Athens Journal of Health* 1: pp. 47–62.

Okay ES (2016). *Healing in Motion: The Influence of Locotherapy on the Architecture of the Pergamene Asklepieion in the second century.* Los Angeles: University of California. https://escholarship.org/uc/item/8sp373gm.

Ottaway P (2004). *Roman York.* Stroud: Tempus.

Oxtoby K (2016). Is the Hippocratic Oath still relevant to practising doctors today? *British Medical Journal* 355: pp. 2–4.

Panagiotidou O (2016). Religious healing and the Asclepius cult: A case of placebo effects. *Open Theology* 2: pp. 79–91.

Papavramidou N and Christopoulou-Aletra H (2009). Medicinal use of leeches in the texts of ancient Greek, Roman and early Byzantine writers. *Internal Medicine Journal* 39: pp. 624–627.

Parker HT (1997). Women doctors in Greece, Rome and the Byzantine Empire, in LR Furst (ed.). *Women Healers and Physicians: Climbing a Long Hill.* Lexington: University Press of Kentucky, pp. 143–162.

Pellegrino ED and Pellegrino AA (1988). Humanism and ethics in Roman medicine: Translation and commentary on a text of Scribonius Largus. *Literature and medicine* 7: pp. 22–38.

Pellegrino ED (2006). Toward a reconstruction of medical morality. *The American Journal of Bioethics* 6: pp. 65–71.

Penn RG (1994). *Medicine on Ancient Greek and Roman Coins*. London: Batsford.

Pérez AB (2018). *Gordian III and the Imperial Petition of Skaptopara*. http://www.judaism-and-rome.org/gordian-iii-and-imperial-petition-skaptopara.

Perlman AI, Ali A, Njike VY, *et al.* (2012) Massage therapy for osteoarthritis of the knee: A randomized dose-finding trial. *PLoS ONE* 7: e30248. https://doi.org/10.1371/journal.pone.0030248

Petridou G (2016). Healing shrines, in GL Irby (ed.). *A Companion to Science, Technology, and Medicine in Ancient Greece and Rome*. Chichester: John Wiley, pp. 434–449.

Petrovska BB (2012). Historical review of medicinal plants' usage. *Pharmacognosy reviews* 6: pp. 1–5.

Photos-Jones E and Hall AJ (2014). Lemnian earth, alum and astringency: A field-based approach, in D Michaelides (ed.). *Medicine and Healing in the Ancient Mediterranean World*. Oxford: Oxbow Books, pp. 183–189.

Photos-Jones E (2018). From mine to apothecary: An archaeo-biomedical approach to the study of the Greco-Roman lithothera-peutics industry. *World Archaeology* 50: pp. 418–433.

Popkin ML (2018). Urban images in glass from the late Roman Empire: The souvenir flasks of Puteoli and Baiae. *American Journal of Archaeology* 122: pp. 427–462.

Powell O (2003). *Galen: On the Properties of Foodstuffs*. Cambridge: Cambridge University Press.

Price E (2000). *Frocester: A Romano-British Settlement, Its Antecedents and Successors*. Stonehouse: Gloucester and District Archaeological Research Group.

Prioreschi P (1998). *Roman Medicine*. Omaha, Nebraska: Horatius Press.

Putnam, B. (1997). The Dorchester Roman aqueduct. *Current Archaeology* 154: pp. 364–369.

Radice B (1963). *The Letters of the Younger Pliny*. London: Penguin.

Ratcliffe JF (2013). *The De Medicina, Cornelius Celsus and Surgery in the First Century CE (Doctoral Thesis)*. Queensland: University of Queensland.

Reilly S, Nolan C, Monckton L (2018). *Wellbeing and the Historic Environment*. London: Historic England.

Rémy B (1984). Les Inscriptions de Médecins en Gaule. *Gallia* 42: pp. 115–152.

Roberts C and Cox M (2003). *Health and Disease in Britain. From Prehistory to the Present Day*. Stroud: Sutton.

Robertson D (2010). *The Philosophy of Cognitive-Behavioural Therapy (CBT)*. London: Karnac.

Robertson D (2019). *How to think like a Roman Emperor. The Stoic Philosophy of Marcus Aurelius*. New York: St Martin's Press.

Rocca J (2008). Anatomy, in RJ Hankinson (ed.). *The Cambridge Companion to Galen*. Cambridge: Cambridge University Press, pp. 242–262.

Rose G (1992). *The Strategy of Preventive Medicine*. Oxford: Oxford University Press.

Rothenhöfer P (2018). Mantias – An eye doctor of the Emperor Tiberius. *Gephyra* 15: pp. 191–195.

Rotherham ID (2012). *Roman Baths in Britain*. Stroud: Amberley.

Rowan E (2014). *Roman Diet and Nutrition in the Vesuvian Region: A Study of the Bioarchaeological Remains from the Cardio V Sewer at Herculaneum*. DPhil (Doctor of Philosophy) thesis, University of Oxford.

Royal College of Surgeons, Professional Standards (2019). *Surgical Innovation, New Techniques and Technologies*. London: Royal College of Surgeons.

Sackett DL, Rosenberg WMC, Muir Gray JA, *et al.* (1996). Evidence based medicine: What it is and what it isn't. *British Medical Journal* 312: pp. 71–72.

St John PD and Montgomery PR (2014). Utility of Hippocrates' prognostic aphorism to predict death in the modern era: Prospective cohort study. *British Medical Journal* 349: pp. 46–47.

Scarborough J (1969). *Roman Medicine*. London: Thames and Hudson.

Scarborough J (1996). Drugs and medicines in the Roman world. *Expedition Magazine* 38.2: pp. 38–51.

Scarth HM (1880). On an inscribed votive tablet found at Binchester (the Ancient Vinovium), Co. Durham in 1879. *Archaeological Journal* 37: pp. 129–135.

Schoenborn NL, Bowman TL, Cayea, D, *et al.* (2016). Primary care practitioners' views on incorporating long-term prognosis in the care of older adults. *JAMA Internal Medicine* 176: pp. 671–678.

Scobie A (1986). Slums, sanitation, and mortality in the Roman world. *KLIO* 68: pp. 399–433.

Scott SP (1932). *The Civil Law*. Cincinnati: The Central Trust Company.

Scott SR, Shafer MM, Smith KE, *et al.* (2020). Elevated lead exposure in Roman occupants of Londinium: New evidence from the archaeological record. *Archaeometry* 62: pp. 109–129.

Shakespeare W (2007 ed.) *Hamlet (Penguin Classics)*. London: Penguin.

Siegel RE (1976). *Galen on the Affected Parts*. Basel: Karger.

Simmonds A, Márquez-Grant N, Loe L (2008). *Life and Death in a Roman City. Excavation of a Mass Grave at 120–122 London Road, Gloucester*. Oxford: Oxford Archaeological Unit.

Singer PN (1997). *Galen: Selected Works*. Oxford: Oxford University Press.

Singer PN (ed.) (2013). *Galen. Psychological Writings*. Cambridge: Cambridge University Press.

Soga M, Gaston KJ, Yamaura Y (2017). Gardening is beneficial for health: A meta-analysis. *Preventive Medicine Reports* 5: pp. 92–99.

Soutelo SG (2014). Medicine and spas in the Roman period: The role of doctors in establishments with mineral-medicinal waters, in D Michaelides (ed.). *Medicine and Healing in the Ancient Mediterranean World.* Oxford: Oxbow Books, pp. 206–216.

Spencer WG (1971). *Celsus: De Medicina (Loeb Classical Library).* Cambridge, MA: Harvard University Press.

Stacey RJ (2011). The composition of some Roman medicines: Evidence for Pliny's punic wax? *Anal Bioanal Chem.* 401: pp. 1749–1759.

Staniforth M (1964). *Marcus Aurelius: Meditations.* London: Penguin.

Stensvold D, Viken H, Steinshamn SL, *et al.* (2020). Effect of exercise training for five years on all cause mortality in older adults – the Generation 100 study: Randomised controlled trial. *BMJ* 371: m3485.

Stephens GR (1985a). Civic aqueducts in Britain. *Britannia* 16: pp. 197–207.

Stephens GR (1985b). Military aqueducts in Roman Britain. *Archeol J.* 142: pp. 216–236.

Stephens JC (2012). The dreams of Aelius Aristides: A psychological interpretation. *International Journal of Dream Research* 5: pp. 76–86.

Stewart EA, Shuster LT, Rocca WA (2012). Reassessing hysterectomy. *Minnesota Medicine* 95: pp. 36–39.

Sturm VE, Datta S, Roy AR, *et al.* (2020). Big smile, small self: Awe walks promote prosocial positive emotions in older adults. *Emotion*: https://doi.org/10.1037/emo0000876.

Summerton N (1999). *Diagnosing Cancer in Primary Care.* Abingdon: Radcliffe.

Summerton N (2000). Trends in negative defensive medicine within general practice. *Br J Gen Pract.* 50: pp. 565–566.

Summerton N (2007). *Medicine and Health Care in Roman Britain.* Princes Risborough: Shire Archaeology.

Summerton N (2011). *Primary Care Diagnostics.* Abingdon: Radcliffe.

Summerton N (2013). Reconstructing ancient medical remedies. *ARA News* 30: pp. 28–30.

Summerton N (2015). Reconstructing a brass box for Roman eye medicines. *ARA News* 34: pp. 38–40.

Summerton N (2018). *Better Value Health Checks: A Practical Guide.* Abingdon: CRC Press.

Taylor SC (2007). *The Bare Necessities? A Comparative Study of the Material Evidence for Roman Medical Practice in Urban Domestic and Army Spheres (MPHIL Thesis).* St Andrews: University of St Andrews.

Temkin O (1956). *Soranus' Gynaecology.* Baltimore: Johns Hopkins.

Tester-Jones M, White MP, Elliott LR, *et al.* (2020). Results from an 18 country cross-sectional study examining experiences of nature for people with common mental health disorders. *Sci Rep* 10: 19408. https://doi.org/10.1038/s41598-020-75825-9.

Thomas JM, Cooney LM, Fried TR (2019). Prognosis reconsidered in light of ancient insights – From Hippocrates to modern medicine. *JAMA Intern Med.* 179: pp. 820–823.

Thomas PH (1963). Graeco-Roman medical and surgical instruments; with special reference to Wales and the border. *J Coll. Gen. Pract.* 6: pp. 495–502.

Tick E (2001). *The Practice of Dream Healing. Bringing Ancient Greek Mysteries into Modern Medicine.* Wheaton: Quest Books.

Tomlin RSO (1991). Inscriptions. *Britannia* 22: pp. 292–311.

Tong TYN, Wareham NJ, Khaw KT, *et al.* (2016). Prospective association of the Mediterranean diet with cardiovascular disease incidence and mortality and its population impact in a non-Mediterranean population: The EPIC-Norfolk study. *BMC Med* 14: 135. https://doi.org/10.1186/s12916-016-0677-4.

Tosh J (2010). *The Pursuit of History.* London: Pearson.

Totelin L (2015). When foods become remedies in ancient Greece: The curious case of garlic and other substances. *Journal of Ethnopharmacology* 167: pp. 30–37.

Touwaide A (2014). Compound medicines in Antiquity: A first approach, in D Michaelides (ed.). *Medicine and Healing in the Ancient Mediterranean World*. Oxford: Oxbow Books, pp. 167–182.

Toynbee JMC (1971). *Death and Burial in the Roman World*. London: Thames and Hudson.

Tullo E (2010). Trepanation and Roman medicine: A comparison of osteoarchaeological remains, material culture and written texts. *The Journal of the Royal College of Physicians of Edinburgh* 40: pp. 165–171.

Ulrich RS (1984). View through a window may influence recovery from surgery. *Science* 224: pp. 420–421.

Ulrich RS (2016). Evidence-based health-care architecture. *Lancet* 368: pp. 538–539.

Vallance JT (1990). *The Lost Theory of Asclepiades of Bithynia*. Oxford: Clarendon Press.

van der Ploeg GE (2016). *The Impact of the Roman Empire on the Cult of Asclepius. A Thesis Submitted for the Fulfilment of the Requirements for the Degree of Doctor of Philosophy in Classics and Ancient History University of Warwick*. University of Warwick: Department of Classics and Ancient History. http://wrap.warwick.ac.uk/79956.

van Tellingen C (2007). Pliny's pharmacopoeia or the Roman treat. *Netherlands Heart Journal* 15: pp. 118–120.

Vauthey M and Vauthey P (1983). Les ex-voto anatomiques de la Gaule romaine (Essai sur les maladies et infirmités de nos ancêtres) – Chapitre IV. *Revue archéologique du Centre de la France* 22–2: pp. 75–81.

Vogt S (2008). Drugs and pharmacology, in RJ Hankinson (ed.). *The Cambridge Companion to Galen*. Cambridge: Cambridge University Press, pp. 304–322.

Voinot J (1999). *Les cachets à collyres dans le monde romain (Monographies instrumentum 7)*. Montagnac: M Mergoil.

Volpp KG, Loewenstein G, Asch DA (2012). Choosing wisely: Low-value services, utilization, and patient cost sharing. *JAMA* 308: pp. 1635–1636.

Wacher J (1995). *The Towns of Roman Britain*. Abingdon: Routledge.

Wallace-Hadrill A (1986). *Ammianus Marcellinus: The Later Roman Empire (AD 354–378)*. London: Penguin.

Waller OH (ed.) (1971). Medicines of Roman Times. *Pharmaceutical Historian* 2: pp. 3–4.

Walters B (2009). Roman villas in Britain: Farms, temples or tax-depots? *Current Archaeology* 230: pp. 30–35.

Wargocki P (2013). The effects of ventilation in homes on health. *International Journal of Ventilation* 12: pp. 101–118.

Watson NM, Wells TJ, Cox C (1998). Rocking chair therapy for dementia patients: Its effect on psychosocial well-being and balance. *American Journal of Alzheimer's Disease* 13: pp. 296–308.

Wellesley K (1972). *Tacitus: The Histories*. London: Penguin.

Wells C (1967). A Roman surgical instrument from Norfolk. *Antiquity* 41: pp. 139–141.

Wheeler REM and Wheeler TV (1932). *Report on the Excavation of the Prehistoric, Roman, and Post-Roman Site in Lydney Park, Gloucestershire*. London: The Society of Antiquaries.

White RH and Barker P (1998). *Wroxeter. Life and Death of a Roman City*. Stroud: Tempus.

Whitmore AM (2013). *Small Finds and the Social Environment of the Roman baths*. PhD (Doctor of Philosophy) thesis, University of Iowa. https://doi.org/10.17077/etd.tr4qgl2i.

Wightman EM (1970). *Roman Trier and the Treveri*. London: Hart-Davis.

Williams T (2003). Water and the Roman city: Life in Roman London, in P Wilson (ed.). *The Archaeology of Roman Towns: Studies in Honour of John S. Wacher*. Oxford: Oxbow Books, pp. 242–250.

Wright RP (1964). A Graeco-Egyptian amulet from a Romano-British site at Welwyn, Herts. *The Antiquaries Journal* 44: pp. 143–146.

Wright RP (1985). A revised restoration of the inscription on the mosaic pavement found in the temple at Lydney Park, Gloucestershire. *Britannia* 16: pp. 248–249.

Yegül F (2010). *Bathing in the Roman World.* Cambridge: Cambridge University Press.

Index